THE GIFT OF OUR

Compulsions

THE GIFT OF OUR

Compulsions

A Revolutionary Approach to
Self-Acceptance and Healing

MARY O'MALLEY

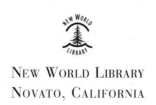

NEW WORLD LIBRARY
NOVATO, CALIFORNIA

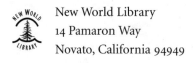

New World Library
14 Pamaron Way
Novato, California 94949

Front cover design by Mary Ann Casler
Text design and typography by Tona Pearce Myers

Library of Congress Cataloging-in-Publication Data
O'Malley, Mary.
  The gift of our compulsions : a revolutionary approach to self-acceptance and healing / Mary O'Malley.— 1st ed.
    p.   cm.
Includes bibliographical references and index.
ISBN 1-57731-470-0 (pbk. : alk. paper)
1. Compulsive behavior. 2. Self-acceptance. 3. Healing. I. Title.
RC533.O436 2004
616.85'84—dc22   2004011494

First printing, October 2004
ISBN 1-57731-470-0

 Printed in Canada on 100% postconsumer waste recycled paper

 A proud member of the Green Press Initiative

Distributed to the trade by Publishers Group West

10   9   8   7   6   5   4   3   2   1

This book is dedicated to the wellspring of deep wisdom in us all. May each of us discover its truth, living from its clarity, love, and support. In this living, the world will be healed.

Contents

Part Four
Treasure Hunting

Acknowledgments

A book is a living process funneled through the mind and heart of the author, with much assistance from many different directions. This was certainly true in the creation of this book. So many wonderful, committed, and inspired people supported its birth, and they have my deep gratitude for the parts they played:

MarySue Phillips: the midwifery of your deep wisdom and your unfailing commitment to this work is appreciated beyond words.

Virginia Howell: your feedback took this book to a whole new level. Thank you for being there in so many ways.

Vaughan and Lyn Mason: this book wouldn't have happened without your support in ways that are too numerous to mention.

Nancy Murray: your razor-sharp ability to cut the superfluous parts in a way I could handle is amazing! I am so glad we are together in this life.

Nancy Hutto, Barb Yamasaki, and Dee Smethurst: your sharp eyes and understanding of language, along with your resonance with the heart of this book, brought it to a higher level of clarity and professionalism.

The Compulsion Groups: the feedback you gave after reading the first draft was invaluable, and I am so thankful you are all in my life.

Mark Ricker and Patrick Hill: you kept me up and running when the world of computers brought me to my knees!

Mimi Kusch, my manuscript editor at New World Library: to work with an editor as skilled as you was pure joy. Through your insight and expertise you simplified, clarified, and enhanced this book. My heart says thank you.

Kristen Cashman, managing editor at New World Library: I feel gratitude for your willingness to walk with me though all the ups and downs of birthing this book. It is a much better book because of your input. Many thanks for being there.

And to all the people who have read parts of this book, adding their perspective in the process, thank you!

Introduction

To some degree, we are all compulsive. By compulsive, I mean engaging in any recurring activity to manage our feelings, an activity that eventually ends up managing us. We can get compulsive in many different ways — by overspending, overeating, overworking, overplanning, overworrying, overexercising, overdrinking, overcomputerizing, or just "overovering." Many of us are compulsive without even knowing it. It isn't until the computer crashes or the credit card is canceled or the doctor says we can't eat a high-fat diet that it becomes clear just how much a particular activity controls our lives.

Ultimately, our core compulsion is to struggle. We live in a story in our heads that is always trying to get us to "do" life, telling us we need to make ourselves and our lives better or different from what they are. In our endless trying, we have forgotten the awesome power of simply paying attention to what we are experiencing in this moment. We have forgotten how to *be*. We have also forgotten how to trust ourselves, to trust our lives, and to live in joy. So we turn to our compulsions to numb ourselves out from all our struggles, only to find ourselves struggling with our compulsions.

It is possible to move beyond struggle and instead reconnect with the joy, wonder, and vitality of being truly alive. This type of healing doesn't just mean that our compulsions would no longer overtake our lives; rather, I mean that we would again be able to experience the deep peace that comes from being comfortable in our own skins, knowing that we are okay, that life is okay, and that everything is going to be okay.

What we will be exploring together in this book is a new approach to working with compulsions that not only heals our compulsions but also allows us to be healed to our core. My life is a testimony to the fact that this is possible. At one time, I gained ninety-seven pounds in a year! Working with the principles and practices put forth in this book, I awakened out of endless struggle into a dynamic, healing, and harmonious relationship with life and the challenges it brings. I have been sharing all that I have learned with others for more than twenty years as an author, counselor, and public speaker.

To heal in this way, we need to learn how to be in a new type of relationship with our compulsions. We have been taught to dominate them, only to have them dominate us. And if we do control one, another seems to take us over. We stop smoking, and we find ourselves overeating. We let go of drinking, and we end up shopping. We try to think positive thoughts to stop our worrying, and we find our to-do lists taking over our lives.

When we try to control our compulsions we think that this will hold back these powerful urges, *but controlling never brings us the lasting healing that we long for.* Instead, it actually fuels the compulsive cycle. It has been widely reported that 95 to 98 percent of all the weight that is lost in the United States is gained back within a year and a half! In fact, people usually gain back more weight than they lost. What we fight controls us. What we resist persists.

There is another way of working with compulsions, a way that will bring us home to ourselves, helping us to open what has been closed, to reclaim what has been hidden, and to remember what has been forgotten. This new way moves us beyond seeing our compulsions as enemies needing to be conquered to recognizing them as guides back into a deep and abiding relationship with ourselves and our lives. This new way is about being *curious* rather than *controlling* and about *responding* rather than *reacting.* Our compulsions thrive in reaction. They heal in response. They won't let go until they teach us how to engage with them, giving them the attention and the compassion they need to heal. In the light of our compassionate attention, not only do our compulsions lose their power over us, but they also become a doorway into the healing that we long for.

To learn the art of being curious rather than reactive, in this book we will be exploring what could be called alchemy. In the Middle Ages, it was thought that alchemy was about turning base metals into gold. Some people believed this so deeply that they spent their lives pursuing this fantasy. True alchemy is much more powerful than that. It is about using the light of human attention to transform the dense, dark clouds of our forgetting into the aliveness and joy of our remembering. As I describe in greater detail in my first book, *Belonging to Life*,[1] it is about cultivating curiosity and compassion in order to transform the holdings in our minds, bodies, and hearts back into the free-flowing aliveness that we truly are.

In part 1 we look at what we are truly longing for whenever we are compulsive. In part 2 we explore how our compulsions have served us. We then explore the difference between our old style of working with compulsions — endlessly trying to manage them — and the new style we are learning, which is about engaging with them so that we can listen, learn, and make skillful choices. In part 3 we cultivate four skills using this new style, allowing us to heal and be healed by our compulsions. Each chapter in this part is devoted to a particular skill. The first skill, Cultivating Curiosity, takes us beyond our ideas of what should be so that we can simply experience what we are experiencing. Using the second skill, Loving Ourselves from the Inside Out, we meet ourselves from the spaciousness of our hearts. We use the third skill, Opening to Our Breath, to nourish and inspire ourselves with the wisdom of our breath. We then apply the fourth skill, Coming Home to Ourselves, to invite ourselves back into our bodies and into a deep and abiding relationship with ourselves and with the present moment — what we are truly longing for whenever we are compulsive. At the end of each of these chapters, I have included a "practices" section to help you apply the skills you have learned.

Finally, in part 4 we bring everything we have explored so far into four questions that we can use in our healing. First we apply these questions to the sensations in our bodies, then to our feelings, and then to our compulsions themselves. These questions are designed to dissolve the core patterns in our minds, to open our hearts to healing, and to put us in direct contact with the wellspring of deep knowing within us that will guide us home.

Throughout the book I have included stories, exercises, and meditations to help you work through particular issues, and every chapter ends with a "Core Ideas" section to help you focus on the ideas presented in that chapter. Working with all these tools will bring us the deep healing we long for, opening us to the truth that we are not alone. Help is always available from our own inner wisdom, which is connected to the wisdom at the heart of life. As we make contact with our wisdom, we have the capacity to let go of *doing* life and we *become* life instead, reconnecting with the healing of simply *being*. I have also included an appendix that provides a handy reference guide to all the skills and techniques explored in the book and a list of resources, including the titles of many wonderful books that I hope you will find useful on your path to healing.

As we allow our compulsions to be a guide back to ourselves, not only will we be healed, but we will also become part of the healing of our planet. When we learn how to listen to our compulsions, they will teach us how to be conscious, compassionate, loving, wise human beings. Living from our inner wellspring of wisdom, we will find ourselves relating to our friends, our family, and all the people we meet from a wiser, more compassionate place. And then, no matter where we are or what is happening in our lives, we become a healing presence in the world.

THE GIFT OF OUR

Compulsions

PART ONE

THE HEALING

Journey

Chapter 1

MY JOURNEY, OUR

Journey

I trust myself. How long has it been since you have been able to say this? Take a moment and imagine what it would be like to really trust yourself. Trusting yourself is about loving yourself from the inside out, accepting every part of your being. It is about living in your body, connected to an inner wellspring of deep wisdom that supports and guides you every moment of your life. And it is about having a responsive mind, one that is passionately curious about what is happening right here, right now.

I also trust my life.

I know how to wake up each morning and open to the unfolding of my day — both the easy and the difficult parts of it — aware that whatever shows up is a part of my journey into an ever-deepening connection with life. I am much more fascinated with showing up for *what is* than with trying to make it into what I think it *should be*. The joy this brings is beyond words.

How have I been fortunate enough to find a deep and wondrous connection with myself and with life when so many people live in reaction, existing in a world of struggle that is usually subtle and sometimes very painful? So many live in the belief that they need to be better or different from what they are to be okay. How do I experience a deep love affair with myself when so many not only do not love themselves but think that if they do they are being selfish? And how did I discover the joy of living in my body when so many live almost exclusively in their heads, believing that their bodies are just vehicles for maneuvering through their lives rather than wellsprings of wisdom, clarity, and support? The amazing thing is that it was my compulsions that brought me to a deep and abiding connection with myself and with life.

It wasn't always that way. As a child I lived in a household where nobody was really there, a familiar experience for many of us. Sure, people were going through the motions of living, but there was no real human contact. There were no playful eyes, no loving arms, no listening hearts that welcomed me into the world and let me know that I was valued for who I was. Children need a sense of connection and support from their caregivers. Being deprived of this essential nutrient of life, I left the world of *I am!*, in which I was easily and comfortably myself, and instead based my life on the belief that *I am not/I should be* — that I was not smart enough, beautiful enough, witty enough, that I had to change myself to make myself "better." I became a human *doing* rather than a human *being*, and the further I got away from who I really was, the more I lived from fear. I tried to make myself into the right kind of person to get the connection that I so desperately needed, but it was never enough.

By the time I was a teenager, self-judgment and despair filled me to my core, and my life became a never-ending maze of pain. I became vulnerable to anything that promised to make me feel better — and compulsions topped the list. I discovered that they could temporarily free me from the deep unease, struggle, and heartache that made up my inner life. When my cravings were satiated, I could relax all my trying, and for brief moments, I could taste a bit of the deep joy I had known before I had disconnected from myself. But quickly the self-hate and despair (that always came after a wave of compulsive activity) would devour my peace, and I would tumble back into that familiar place of struggle.

For almost half my life, I both hated my compulsions and desperately needed them in order to survive. They numbed my heartache enough so that I could at least function. I was taught that my compulsions were bad, and yet they relieved the pressure of always trying to make myself better or different from what I was. Binging on food is one of the strongest memories of my childhood, as I desperately tried to ingest the love I craved. I can remember when I was twelve years old, coming home from school, putting two pieces of toast in the toaster, and as soon as they popped up, putting in two more. Quickly buttering the finished toast, I stuffed them into my mouth so that I would be ready to butter and eat the next two. On and on I went until the fullness in my stomach temporarily numbed the emptiness in my heart.

I then went on to discover the mind-numbing world of prescription drugs, alcohol, busyness, and even some street drugs. Over time, most of these habits dropped away, but my core compulsion — overeating — remained. My descent into eating hell took many twists and turns over the years, all accompanied by great self-hatred, deep despair, and a sinking feeling that I was just too weak-willed to take control. Every failure at being in charge only fueled more self-disgust, which brought on more eating. After years of failed diets, counseling, shots, pills, hypnosis clinics, fasting, and anything else that promised a way out of this descending spiral, I weighed 220 pounds. I, like everyone else, was trying to heal my compulsion using the only method that was around at that time — *control.*

Learning to Listen

Thank God that controlling my compulsion didn't work for me. Stripped of any illusion that I was powerful enough to be in charge of these deep forces that would come roaring through me, I began to hear, as if over a very fuzzy phone line, a deep knowing inside me. This knowing said that lasting healing comes from being curious rather than controlling, that it comes from mercy rather than manipulation, from responding rather than reacting. It is about opening what has been closed, reclaiming what has been hidden, and remembering what has been forgotten.

I began to work with a woman who deeply understood these truths, and like a comet returning from the depths of outer space, I began the journey back to myself. One of the first things she invited me to do was to let go of the violence of dieting. This was like asking me to jump off the end of the world. I just knew that I would gain a thousand pounds in a month. But after a small weight gain, things began to settle down. As the clouds of my controlling mind began to lift a little, I could see that it was in listening to what was going on inside me when I was compulsive, rather than living in the endless cycles of reaction, that I would be healed.

So I began to listen.

Even though the compulsive eater within me would still rage through my life, leaving great devastation in its wake, I was becoming curious about what exactly was going on when I wanted to overeat. Slowly and surely, rather than hating my compulsion, I began to feel a bit of respect for it. Watching it in action, I realized that it was an old survival tool that I had picked up when I was young. I truly believed that if I ignored, denied, or ran away from anything unpleasant in my life, everything would be okay. When I finally began to truly listen, I could see not only that this did not work, but also that the exact opposite was happening. When I felt anxiety, I would numb out by overeating, and then I would feel more fear. (I will never be able to control myself, and I will just get fatter!) When I felt self-judgment, I would overeat, and then I would feel deep shame. (You are such a failure for not being able to control yourself!)

Noticing that my compulsions never brought me the deep peace I longed for and that trying to control them only made them worse, I began to become truly curious. Even just a few moments of being curious when a wave of compulsion arrived dramatically lessened my compulsive urges, and for years these bouts of uncontrolled eating lessened. *I was no longer fighting them, so they weren't fighting me.* My body discovered the weight it was comfortable at, and I ate mostly what I wanted, when I wanted. I can still remember the first autumn when sweets didn't look interesting. All the soccer candy, Girl Scout cookies, and Halloween junk didn't capture my attention. I was amazed!

There were times when the urge to eat everything in sight — and then some — would return, but it was more like a big ocean wave passing through than the devastation of a tsunami. Sometimes I could be curious for a moment or two while the wave of compulsion was passing through, but most of the time I could not bring any curiosity to bear until the wave had stopped. Even though I had received so much healing from learning how not to fight my compulsion, I hadn't yet learned how to meet and explore all the hidden feelings that fueled my periodic binges.

That was soon to change. After a number of glorious years of being in balance with food, my health began to deteriorate in my late thirties. My doctors suggested some fairly heavy dietary restrictions, and I began to re-experience all the feelings that were frozen inside me from being on a restricted diet when I was young. I had been born highly allergic to wheat, eggs, chocolate, and dairy products. If you think about it for a moment, you will realize that I couldn't eat "kid food" — no birthday cakes, cookies, hot dogs, sandwiches, or Hershey bars. In other words, I was always on the outside looking in, whether it was at birthday parties, the school cafeteria, or eating with my family. This created feelings of isolation, rage at being left out, and a sense that something was wrong with me. These feelings were a core part of my childhood and a hidden part of my adulthood. I finally rebelled as a teenager and had been eating unskillfully since then.

Now the doctors were telling me I had to go back to the food restrictions of my childhood! The compulsive eater inside me woke up and was having none of this. It didn't want to experience again all those agonizing feelings that come from a severely limited choice of foods. When I was told that wheat was poison to my body and that I should never eat it again, I went out and ate lots and lots of wheat — toast, cookies, whatever.

In reaction, I desperately tried to hold on to control, even though I knew somewhere deep inside me that it would only make matters worse. This time I didn't use diets. Instead I used eating programs whose focus was about health rather than weight loss. My intent in following these programs was more benevolent than my previous intent to lose weight. Yet I still was looking to somebody else's ideas about how I should eat rather than learning how to listen to myself. I hadn't yet discovered that only my body can tell me what I need to maintain balance and health.

After experiencing again the devastation of trying to control these urges only to have them control me, my curiosity kicked in again. I could now see that my core compulsion was to struggle, and my other compulsions had all been an attempt to numb out from the chaos, confusion, and despair that came from struggling. So rather than struggling with my compulsions, which only created more struggle, I began to listen when the old urges would come. I began to listen so deeply that I was able to see what I was trying to run away from when I was compulsive. And (big surprise!) all the feelings of being left out, defective, and hopeless that had been buried deep inside me since I was young were there when I wanted to binge. I could finally recognize *why* I was overeating. This was pay dirt.

I began to develop a relationship with the feelings that were fueling my eating binges. What I was doing with these feelings was probably different from anything I had tried before. I wasn't so much *feeling* these feelings as I was *meeting* them. There is a huge difference between these two things. In *feeling* a feeling you can get lost in the middle of it. *Meeting* a feeling is about relating *to* the feeling, giving it the attention and understanding it needs to be transformed back into free-flowing energy. As I met each of the old, frozen feelings that were fueling these binges, meeting them with my compassionate attention, they lost their power over me.

Through this willingness to listen to my compulsion and the feelings it was trying to manage, my compulsive eater and I became partners in my healing. When I committed to being *present for* my compulsion in a nonviolent way, it showed me all the parts of me that needed the healing of my curious and compassionate heart. As I met my feelings, I no longer needed to numb myself. Overeating became less and less a part of my life, as more and more parts of me became healed through my compassionate attention.

Being Present for Yourself

If you have ever been taken over by something that you cannot control — whether it is overeating, overdrinking, overspending, overworrying, or overworking — you will understand the intense gratitude I felt in learning how to come back into balance. At the time, I believed that was the extent of my healing. Little did I know that I had just begun to taste the joy of coming back to myself. As I became more able to be present for myself during a wave of compulsion, I began to be present at other times as well. Instead of that heavy, constantly struggling mode of existence I had lived in most of my life, I began to feel lighter. The tiny flicker of joy that used to be hidden deep inside me began to grow into a flame and then eventually into a warm and toasty fire that warmed me from my core.

I was becoming myself — not an idea of what I should be, not an ongoing project that always needed to be better or different, but truly and authentically myself. I was moving into a place of pure being — alive, joyous, trusting, and full of love. I was connected to an inner wellspring of deep knowing that supported and guided me. I finally saw that it was never food that I was hungry for. Rather, what I was really longing for was a deep and abiding relationship with who I truly am. This concept felt totally new to me, for even though all children know a rudimentary form of this kind of connection when they are young, as an adult I have no memories of it. Very early on I had lost connection with myself, pulling myself up and out of my body and becoming lost in my head. Being that disconnected, I lost trust in myself and in life. I had even lost the knowing that I had lost anything!

Being present for my compulsion helped me to meet all the parts of myself I had rejected, taking me step-by-step back into wholeness I had never known. I no longer live in a mind at war with itself. I know the joy of loving myself from the inside out, and being connected to my body again puts me in contact with the wellspring of joy and wisdom that resides there. Every once in a while I still get scared and my compulsion looks interesting, but in a very gentle way. And because these little waves of compulsion always take me another step into a deeper connection with myself and with life, now I even trust them.

I am telling you this story because it isn't mine alone. I am not just one of the lucky few who have healed and been healed by their compulsions. More and more of us have learned all that we can from trying to manage our compulsions, finally realizing that controlling them will never bring us the deep healing we long for. We are now ready for the next step — to heal and be healed by our compulsions. We are also beginning to comprehend that it is our birthright to make the journey back home — back to ourselves, back to our essence, which is the wellspring of joy, peace, creativity, and trust within us. The wonderful thing is that this type of healing, reclaiming the truth of who you really are, doesn't affect just you. As you heal yourself, you heal the world. For the mind-set that fuels our compulsions and then fights with what it has created is the same mind-set that has caused such heartache all over the world. This compulsion to struggle with life shows up in the sense of incompleteness and isolation that is the undercurrent of most people's lives. You can see it in the power games that are the hallmark of most relationships, whether between people, businesses, or countries. It also shows up in the political, religious, and ideological confrontations that are sadly so rampant on our planet.

When we hate and fear our compulsions, and when we judge ourselves for having them, that aggression spills out into our world, adding to the unconsciousness of humanity. When we learn how to be curious and merciful with ourselves and our compulsions, we bring equanimity and kindness to all that we are and do. In this new way of relating to ourselves, we become a part of the healing of this planet.

As more and more of us move beyond our compulsive need to *do* life — always trying to make it be different from what it is — and instead allowing ourselves to *be* life, just like drops of water filling a pond, one day the pond of human consciousness will overflow and the Earth will know the deep peace it longs for. You are reading this book because you are ready to ripen into a full and deep connection with yourself and your life. You are ready to heal at your core and, in that healing, become a part of the healing of our planet.

Let us now explore what took us away from the deep connection with ourselves and what it would be like to return there again.

Core Ideas

- It is your birthright to make the journey back home — back to yourself, back to your essence, which is the wellspring of joy, peace, creativity, and trust within you.

- Trusting yourself is about loving yourself from the inside out, accepting every part of your being. It is about living in your body, connected to an inner wellspring of deep wisdom that supports and guides you every moment of your life. And it is about having a responsive mind, one that is passionately curious about what is happening right here, right now.

- Healing is about becoming yourself — not an idea of what you should be, not an ongoing project that always needs to be better or different, but truly and authentically yourself — alive, joyous, trusting, and full of love.

- Healing is about opening what has been closed, reclaiming what has been hidden, and remembering what has been forgotten.

- Reclaiming the truth of who you really are doesn't affect just you. As you heal yourself, you heal the world. For the mind-set that fuels our compulsions and then fights with what it has created is the same mind-set that has caused such heartache all over the world.

- Compulsions are skillful guides on the journey back home to ourselves.

Chapter 2

RECONNECTING WITH

Yourself

There was a time when you absolutely loved being you. When you were very young you hadn't yet learned how to second-guess yourself. You lived in your body and your heart, and whoever you were was enough. In fact, it was more than enough, *for it was you.* Even if you have no memories of this, your body does. It remembers when you were completely connected to yourself, open to the adventure of life. You felt your enthusiasm for living in every cell of your body, and it was wonderful just to be alive.

All of us — some for a very short time and others for longer — knew this timeless place where we lived in full connection with ourselves and our lives. Before we pulled back from life, we were unshakably attuned to the truth that we were okay, that life was okay, and that everything was going to be okay. Life was a magical adventure. We hadn't yet become caught up in watches and calendars, and nothing was more important than whatever was happening in the moment. We were present for the mischief of a puppy, the magic of the butterfly's dance, and our fascination with having a belly button.

A friend told me a wonderful story of taking a walk through the woods with a three-year-old girl that reveals what it was like for us when we were connected to ourselves and to our lives. Coming to a bridge over a stream, the little girl became completely enamored of the flow of the water, so enamored she had to lie down on the bridge, hanging her head over its edge to see more clearly. Every once in a while she would look up at my friend and simply say, "Wow!" Three times they headed down the path beyond the bridge, and three times the little girl turned around and went back to the wonder of the flowing water. Because she spent no time worrying about who she should be, there were no filters obscuring her pure experience of being alive.

You also knew, as children the world over know, how to keep the joy of life alive by hugging and snuggling, swinging and twirling, dancing and running. Shelby, a friend's three-year-old niece, was at a theater watching a movie full of dancing and singing. There was no way she could sit in her seat! Luckily they happened to be in a row of seats with a space in front of them for a wheelchair. Since that space was not occupied, Shelby danced her way through the movie. When was the last time you felt that kind of vitality and joy?

I hope that these stories have brought up a memory, no matter how faint, of what it was like to love yourself from the inside out, staying open to the magical adventure of your life. Even if you have no memories of your world before all the *shoulds* and *ought-tos* dimmed your love affair with yourself and with life, you too, like all very young children, once enjoyed being authentically *you*. The river of life flowed through you, sometimes in torrents, sometimes in stillness, full of the peace of being connected to life and of being comfortable in your own skin.

This experience was a rudimentary form of the full connection that is possible for you as an adult. When you were young, you were awake to life. As an adult, not only can you be awake, but you can be aware

— curiously and compassionately present. It is possible to wake up in the morning with an abiding love for yourself, a deep appreciation for the gift of life, and a wondrous curiosity about where the adventure is going to take you. Not only is this possible, it is your *birthright.*

Inhabiting the House of Your Being

This ability to be okay with yourself and your life, no matter what is happening, has always been inside you. It may be just a tiny rivulet that you are hardly even aware of, but it is there nonetheless. If you are like most people, you live almost exclusively in a story in your head, and the clouds of thought swirling around keep this deep connection with yourself very well covered. Your thoughts don't eradicate it, but they do cut you off from the nourishment of simply and powerfully being you. As you stay caught in your story of struggle, you are hardly ever aware that just below the thousands of thoughts you pay attention to every day lies another world, one in which you can trust in yourself, trust in life, and feel the joy that is your true nature.

How can it be that we knew such a deep connection with life when we were young, and yet most of the time as adults we find ourselves, on some level, struggling with life and feeling just half-alive? The best way to understand this conundrum is to imagine a glorious house, airy and full of light, with the music of laughter flowing from room to room. This is the house of your *being,* and when you were little, you lived there, fully open. You lived in your body, grounded in the basement of your belly, and the energy of life flowed freely through you. The floors above were the realm of your heart, and all the windows and doors were open to life. Your heart was so alive that with every beat the joy of loving yourself and life was pumped through all the nooks and crannies of your being. And the attic of your mind was a wonderful place of imagination and curiosity, open to the whole house of your being. You were able simply to show up for life's amazing adventure rather than always trying to make it into what you thought it should be.

Because you were so open to life, everything touched you to your core. Remember tasting every bite of your ice cream cone? Remember lying on your back and watching in wonder as the clouds danced for you? Remember the ballet of dust particles, highlighted in the beam of sunlight from your bedroom window?

Basking in the glow of living fully in your body and being in contact with your true nature — when you said, *"I am!"* — that was enough. In fact, it was more than enough, for you were simply and purely yourself. So you didn't need to stop your feelings or run to the illusion of safety in the attic of the mind. During that precious time, there was no part of the house that was off-limits. You hadn't yet come to believe that you needed to be different to receive the nourishment, attention, and connection that you required to survive.

This wouldn't last.

In the openness of your youth, not only were you available to the pure joy of being alive, you were also vulnerable to the actions and expectations of the people around you. The giants in your world (parents, siblings, aunts and uncles, teachers, neighbors, clergy, and a host of others) began to influence you. Life had wounded them, and they passed their wounds on to you. Even if you had parents who loved you, along with what might have looked like a picture-perfect childhood, this wounding still occurred.

Nobody was there meeting you in the place of your wounding, showing you how to stay open to life in the presence of pain. To survive, you learned how to close off parts of yourself, holding your breath and tightening your body. Every time you contracted your body and tried to deny what you were experiencing, you put another part of yourself in a box and hid it in a room in the house of your being. On the door of each room you put a sign that said "Do not open." Underneath those words, in little letters, was the statement "This room is filled with bad feelings." But even though they were behind closed doors, these feelings still influenced your life and eventually fueled your compulsions.

As you grew up and circumstances disappointed, overwhelmed,

confused, and threatened you, you locked more and more rooms of your house. Rather than being airy and filled with light, your house became dark. You were no longer dancing from room to room, and the music of laughter was rarely heard. Soon all the rooms were filled with your boxed-up feelings, so you had to move some of them down into the basement, hoping that they would never torment you again. These were the ones that you were most afraid of — your rage, your terror, and your despair. It was very, very important to keep your belly tight and never to breathe a full breath, for that is how the door to the basement would open again, and you definitely didn't want that to happen.

But all was not lost.

As you were boxing up all your feelings, you were also learning more about the world of thinking. You were discovering what a magical tool it is, but you were also learning that you could hide from life in your thoughts. One day, while exploring the attic of your mind, you discovered a big-screen TV, along with a DVD player and boxes of discs. You found out that you could sit up there and got lost in movies *about* life, which felt a lot safer than actually *experiencing* it. Eventually you found yourself spending more and more time in the attic, especially when experiencing life would have meant dealing with strong and confusing feelings. You left the now curtained and closed-off floors of your body for the tightly enclosed attic of the mind. Because the images in your mind were so compelling, you hardly even noticed that you had lost the true and abiding connection with yourself and with life that you had enjoyed as a child.

The more you lived in your mind, the more you began to truly believe one of its core ideas: "To be safe, you must be in control." Becoming lost in control, you found yourself cut off from your own deep wisdom. Trained to distrust your feelings, you became absolutely certain that you must never go back into the lower floors of the house, especially the basement. Instead you must control, control, control! Gone was the willingness to be open to life. Gone was spontaneous creativity. Gone was the pure joy of being alive.

Even though you may have retained a faint memory of living in the entire house, with all the light and laughter that used to fill it, the movies in your mind were interesting enough to compensate for that, and things stayed fairly balanced for a while. And when they didn't feel balanced, you had your first experience of trying to re-create the joy you knew when you were fully connected to yourself and to life. Maybe it was the glass of wine that turned your body into liquid warmth, the deep relaxation after that first bite of a forbidden food, the joy that came from a buying spree, or even the thrill of winning at gambling. They were faint shadows of the wonderful feelings you had when you inhabited the whole house. But because the whole house was no longer available, those actions seemed adequate substitutes for joy.

Unable to be naturally who you *were,* you began to try to figure out who you *should be,* and there were plenty of DVDs lying around the attic that showed you how to be a successful you. You were so intent on making yourself different from what you were that you didn't notice the voices coming over a loudspeaker in the attic that were critiquing your endless quest for perfection. You also didn't notice that you had left the wonderful world of *I am!* that you knew so well when you were young for the world of *I am not/I should be.*

As the wonderful movies you first watched when you crawled up into the attic gave way to movies full of have-tos, shoulds, and ought-tos, an undercurrent of discontentment, boredom, and quiet despair stirred within you, and you tried very hard not to notice. Since you were cut off from the nourishment of your heart and disconnected from the wellspring of wisdom and support in the basement of your being, your existence in the attic became a constant search for the peace that you knew when you lived in the full house of your whole being. You looked for it in moving on to the next relationship, in spending money, in working out, in gaining a more positive outlook, in driving a fancier car, or in getting a better education. This search took you into classes, therapy, and religion, in the hopes that if you just got yourself in order, everything would be okay.

These activities are fine in and of themselves. But even if you accomplish your goals — if you win the lottery, get your PhD, understand where your pain came from, or learn how to affirm twenty times a day that you are a radiant and peaceful person — *it will never be enough.* There is an essential emptiness that will never be filled by all the doing, accomplishing, and acquiring that are the hallmarks of living in the attic. The deep peace of "enoughness" will only come when you move back into your body and inhabit the entire house of your being.

Opening the Door to Your Feelings

The mind, however, will have nothing to do with moving back into your body, for it remembers how scared it was right before you retreated to the so-called safety of the attic. So in the attic you stayed. Even though things were not all that happy in there, you carried on. One thing, however, upset the careful equilibrium you were trying to establish through control more than anything else — your feelings. You see, *feelings do not like to be boxed up.* They flow from the river of aliveness, and they love to move and dance through your being. Every once in a while, you could hear them demanding attention from the rooms below, but you would just put in another movie and distract yourself again.

You were so busy distracting yourself that you didn't notice that feelings are very crafty and extremely skillful at getting out of the most enclosed spaces. As they learned how to escape from their boxes, they would come pattering up the stairs, knock on the door of the attic, and ask to be let in. But there was a sign on the inside of the door that said "Never, ever open this door! The only safety is in staying in control." And you knew that if you let those feelings in, you would definitely be out of control. So you turned up the volume of the TV.

But feelings don't give up easily, and over time, no matter how far you turned up the volume, you couldn't drown out their persistent knocking. That was when your compulsions, that earlier were just in bud, came into full bloom. It was a sip of wine that turned into glass after glass. It was a cookie that turned into a dozen. Maybe it was a fun night of gambling that turned into a nightmare. It could also be the to-do list that kept getting longer as you frantically ran around trying to get everything done. The deep part of you that just wanted to keep pain at bay discovered that if you gambled, overate, drank, or got overly busy, you could simply ignore all those knocks on your door.

Very quickly the compulsive urge for *more, more, more* turned into *not enough, not enough, not enough.* And after the wave of compulsion moved through, you would be left in self-hatred and despair. No matter how passionately compulsions promised to bring you the peace that you longed for, they never really did. But you didn't know how to stop your compulsions, nor did you know how to get out of the attic and back into what you were truly hungry for — a deep and satisfying connection with yourself and with life. No wonder you had moments — and maybe even weeks, months, and years — when you were depressed and overwhelmed, consumed by a loneliness that nothing could ease.

The more you ran away from these feelings, the more persistent they became and the harder you had to try to keep them at bay, never knowing that the safest thing to do was to open the door, invite them in, and get to know them again. So on you went for years and years, lost in your head, while your feelings knocked at the door and your compulsions tried to keep them at bay. You became even more cut off from yourself when you were taught that compulsions were bad and must be controlled and that if you couldn't control them, *you* were bad. Lost in an ever-increasing battle in the attic of your mind, every once in a while you would hear the sound of the wind outside the attic, and you would get a funny feeling at the core of your being that there was something more to life than the endless reaction and struggle of the attic.

One day you found a dusty DVD that had fallen behind the TV. When you watched it, you realized it was about what it was like when you lived in the whole house. How light and airy it was! You notice such exuberance in your body! There was such a light shining out of your eyes! The longing to be connected again gives you courage. You finally understand that to live in the whole house of your being, you need to *meet* the feelings standing outside the door. The next time you hear one knocking at the door, you decide to listen rather than turning up the TV. What you hear your feelings saying is, "Please don't ignore me. I am a part of you. If you meet me, you can move back into the house of your being, and I will be your friend." It becomes clear that the safest thing to do is to open the door and invite them in for a heart-to-heart talk.

So you open the door just a crack. There are your feelings all standing in a row, waiting to be heard. Immediately you get scared and slam the door shut again. But a wise voice within says this is not about feeling these feelings and getting lost in them again. This is about meeting them, giving them your undivided attention so they can transform back into the free-flowing energy of life. Remembering the DVD about what it was like to live in the whole house, you discover the courage to open the door and invite the first feeling in. You are astounded that the feeling is more afraid of you than you are of it! You ask it to sit down and tell you its story. You listen with rapt attention as it describes how it was born and what it was like all these years to be stuck in the dark and empty rooms of your body.

You realize in a flash that what you have been running from your whole life are very young feelings that you boxed up long ago. And instead of being flawed or defective parts of you, they are just very vulnerable parts that are hurt and afraid and need your help. It finally becomes clear that as long as you run away from them, you will be confined to the attic, cut off from the joy of living in the full house of yourself. As the feeling finishes speaking of its heartache, it goes on to tell you what a joy it was to be a part of you when you were young and how much it would like to be a respected part of you again. You realize with stunning clarity that it is okay to allow this feeling to be a part of you again. With an eagerness you have not experienced in years, you invite another feeling in for a chat, and then another, listening as they tell their stories.

Soon they are inviting you down into the closed rooms of your body, and with joy you begin to unpack all the other boxed-up parts of you. Even though the feelings you find there may be a little grinchy, or even quite scared from being boxed up for so long, you know they are just very young parts of you that need your undivided attention. As you wander through the rooms, opening windows and doors, you begin to remember how wonderful it was when you lived fully in your body. You see everything through new eyes and discover that when you were locked in the attic of your mind, you had forgotten how to be fully alive.

As you become more present, everything calms down and loosens up, and the joy of being alive begins to flow throughout your whole body again. Your shoulders relax, and a smile fills your entire being. The tight band of sadness across your chest begins to loosen, and your breath becomes fuller and easier. The tense fist of endless trying in your stomach starts to let go, and the fear of not being enough begins to melt away. Even the empty hole that your compulsion has never been able to fill becomes a warm glow deep in your belly.

This is the first time since your childhood that you have felt safe enough to open to life, safe enough to be yourself. You realize that whenever you were compulsive, *this is what you were truly hungry for* — a deep and abiding connection with yourself that brings forth the joy of being comfortable in your own skin. Compulsions look less and less interesting to you, for you are being nourished by the joy that comes from living in your body and becoming yourself again — not an idea of what you should be, but the real thing.

As wonderful as it is, you find you can't stay there very long. It is all so new, and sometimes very scary to be this open. So you find yourself retreating back up into the mind and closing the door, especially when strong feelings are moving through you. Sometimes you turn up the TV so you don't have to hear the knocking at the door, and sometimes you even find yourself being compulsive again. But compulsions are now your ally, for you know that whenever you are compulsive, another part of you is standing right outside the locked door asking for your undivided attention. Rather than becoming lost in eating, drinking, or gambling, you are reminded by your compulsions that a part of you needs your understanding attention.

After reclaiming many parts of yourself, there is still one place you have not had the courage to explore — the basement of your belly. This is where you hid the *big* feelings — the monsters of rage, terror, and despair. Everything you have heard about that dark and foreboding place makes you feel that if you ever got the courage even to open the door of the basement, you would be instantly devoured by the monsters from the deep.

Not only are you afraid to go down there, but many of these feelings are very elusive and only seem to surface when your life is in chaos. But you finally understand one of the core functions of compulsion — to highlight these feelings so that they can be healed. So you watch and wait for the next wave, knowing that you are only compulsive when deep feelings are close to the surface. And so with flashlight in hand and heart pounding furiously, you descend to the basement — into the deepest and most tightly held parts of your body — wanting to meet whatever is there.

Much to your amazement, rather than monsters you find the youngest parts of yourself cowering in the corner. They look almost like little wild animals with deep fear in their eyes. Your own fear evaporates as you realize how scared they are. You sit down to reassure them, and say quietly to them, "I'm here. I understand."

It takes them a moment to get over the shock that you were willing to enter the basement (you haven't been there for decades) and the even greater shock that you are willing to talk to them. But hope springs eternal, and in a flash, tears of gratitude begin to roll down their cheeks. With a little coaxing, they come out of the dark corner where they were cowering, and with deep relief crawl into your arms. You find yourself saying to them over and over again, "I'm here now. It's okay; I'm here."

You realize they have been waiting your whole life for you to grow beyond your fear of them so that you could give them exactly what they needed all those years ago — nonjudgmental, loving attention. As you carry them upstairs, they are a little overwhelmed by the rooms filled with light. But as with all young ones, they adapt very quickly. They can be this free, for they know that they are now a valued and accepted part of you. The last of the curtains that held back the light are whisked away, and joyous laughter fills your rooms again.

Every once in a while you feel a wave of compulsion coming on, but rather than reacting to it by retreating to your head, you are able to sit down wherever you are, close your eyes, and breathe all the way into your belly. You can then listen to what you are experiencing there. You have finally awakened enough to take responsibility for your feelings, which is, after all, simply the ability to respond to them. And just a few moments of being with the feelings releases them back into the flow of aliveness that is your birthright, and the wave of compulsion moves through, leaving hardly a trace.

Entering the Circle of Warmth

Looking back over this amazing journey — beginning with the joy of living so fully in your body when you were young, only to lose this connection with yourself, and now finally to rediscover it again — you feel gratitude for how far you have come. But something inside you knows that this journey back to yourself is not yet complete. Sitting quietly one day on your favorite window seat, gazing out on the beauty of nature, you feel compelled to go down to the basement. Since the basement is no longer cluttered with all those scary feelings you so desperately tried to hide there, there is a vast openness that you now experience as joy.

This joy draws you to the very center of the basement where you notice a circular room that was previously hidden by all the boxes of feelings piled around it. When you come close, you realize it is radiating a wonderful warmth, and you know from the deepest part of your *being* that you are supposed to sit down basking in its warmth as you breathe long and slow breaths. As your belly softens and you settle into your body, you become aware of the same kind of warmth glowing inside you. As you open to it, this glow radiates throughout your whole body as waves of light and love fill you from head to toe. When you open your eyes, much to your amazement, the walls of this circular room have dissolved and there before you stands a beautiful spring of burbling water, lush with vibrant green foliage and beautiful flowers.

With deep recognition, you see that this wellspring has always been with you. Its source is the creative forces at the heart of life, the forces that show up as the radiance of the sun, the unfolding of the seasons, and the beating of your heart. You feel an indescribable joy as you kneel beside it and dip your hands in to drink from its essence. As this water flows through your body, you realize that this wellspring is what fills the house of your being with love, light, and the pure joy of being alive. It contains all the elements that truly fulfill you: the fire of the passion for living, the strength of the earth for endurance and perse-verance, the lightness of the air for play and exuberance, the healing quality of water that allows all things to flow, and the love that unites everything.

With great clarity, you understand that your whole life has been a journey toward reconnecting with this inner wellspring. On this jour-ney, you were meant to know the wellspring when you were young, and then leave its healing presence for the long journey into your unique experience of separation. Now it is time to return. You also realize that every part of that journey was necessary. Even though you made many so-called wrong turns, every one of them was a perfect part of the jour-ney away from and then back to yourself. Now, no matter where you are and no matter what is happening, with just one deep breath you can return to this wellspring within and drink your fill.

Finally you understand that you have been given the gift of life because you have risen out of the creativity at the heart of life. *You are one of a kind.* In the vastness of all time, the great and wondrous unfold-ing of life has never ever shown up exactly as you. *Nobody else ever can be a better you than you.* Life is expressing itself as you because it needs to express itself as you. You don't have to figure out what your particu-lar gift is or how to get to it, or even what to do with it. All you need do is drink from this wellspring of wisdom and support that resides at the core of your being. What you are here to do and be will unfold in its own time and its own way. As the last vestiges of tension leave your belly, you feel a sense of deep relief. The old, familiar sense of discontentment gives way to an ease that nourishes you to your core.

You realize that you aren't just one of the lucky few who can know and live from the healing waters of the wellspring within. You see that more and more people are discovering and then living from the integrity, courage, wisdom, and compassion that come from being connected to their own wellsprings. Drinking deeply from its healing waters one more time, you see that you will never again feel alone, for the creative powers at the heart of life are with you and within you. Life will ebb and flow, and you will still live the cycles of remembering and forgetting. But there is no sorrow in this, for you now know the deep peace of *being*. In this knowing, you are willing to show up with a keen, curious mind and a spacious, open heart for whatever life gives you. As you stand again, you realize that finally you are truly yourself. You walk up the stairs and into the unfolding of your life, overflowing with exuberance, curiosity, and the joy of being alive.

It may sound too good to be true, but you can live again in the entire house of your being, connected to your own deep wisdom, trusting of yourself and your life. In fact, that is why this book has come into your life. It is a complete guide to the journey back to you. Everything we will explore together has come out of my own journey, a journey that took me as far away from myself as a human being can go and still survive, a journey that also took me step-by-step back into a full connection with life. As you explore the ideas and do the exercises included in this book, you too can move beyond your compulsions and experience once again a joy-filled connection with the amazing adventure called life.

Core Ideas

• Early on, the river of life flowed through you, sometimes in torrents, sometimes gently, full of the peace of being connected to life and of being comfortable in your own skin.

- When you were very young, the house of your *being* was a wondrous place to explore. There was no part of the house that wasn't okay. Basking in the glow of living fully in your body and being in contact with your true nature — when you said, "*I am!*" — that was enough.

- When life threatened, confused, and disappointed you, you learned how to close off parts of yourself and began to live in the *I am not/I should be* story in your head.

- The more you live in your mind rather than your heart, the more you believe that to be safe you have to be in control, hiding deep within you the spontaneous creativity and pure joy of being alive.

- The deep peace of "enoughness" will only come when you move back into your body and inhabit all the floors of the house of your being. To do this, you need to *meet* the feelings that are standing outside the door of the attic of your mind.

- Meeting your feelings is not about getting lost in them again. It is about giving them your undivided attention so they can transform back into the free-flowing energy of life.

- It is possible to wake up in the morning with an abiding love for yourself, a deep appreciation for the gift of life, and a wondrous curiosity about where the adventure is going to take you. Not only is this possible, it is your *birthright*.

- You have risen out of the creativity at the heart of life. You don't have to figure out what your particular gift is or how to get to it, or even what to do with it. All you need do is drink from the wellspring of wisdom and support that resides at the core of your being. What you are here to do and be will unfold in its own time and its own way.

PART TWO

TRANSFORMING OUR RELATIONSHIP WITH
Compulsions

Chapter 3

RECOGNIZING OUR COMPULSIONS AS

Friends

s we saw in the last chapter, whenever we are compulsive, what
we are really longing for is to reconnect with ourselves. We are
hungry for the experience of being grounded in our bodies
again so we can live from the wellspring within that connects us to
wisdom, to our hearts, and to our lives. This is the connection that we
knew so well when we were young; it has been waiting for us to grow up
enough so that we can know and live it again on an even deeper level.

Compulsions are our guides back into this connection, one that
relaxes our minds, opens our hearts, and brings a twinkle to our eyes.
They are not evidence that you are weak-willed or defective. Rather, they
are powerful forces that are here to heal you to your core. To take this
journey back to ourselves and into our full potential, we need to transform our relationship to our compulsions. If we trace them back to their
roots, it is easy to see that they emerged to help us manage feelings that

were too much for us. As infants, we were completely available to our feelings, both the joyful and the painful ones. The joyful ones kept us connected to our essence. The painful ones caused us to pull back from life. No matter what they were, feelings flowed through us like a river. Imagine yourself as a young child when you read the following scenarios. These may be very familiar to some of us, and to others, they may not. Regardless, they are designed to hint at the multitude of experiences we all had when we were young, many of which caused us to pull back from life:

Exercise

Imagine the exuberance you feel in your body as you yell loudly enough in the grocery store to hear your own echo, only to have an angry clerk grab you from behind and shake you unmercifully; imagine an older sibling stealing your favorite toy and then taunting you with it — the powerless rage you feel is almost too much to bear, even as a memory; imagine the pleasure of playing with your body, only to have a horrified adult face loom above you saying, "Bad, bad, bad!"; imagine being two years old and having a huge dog run toward you while barking fiercely. As you wail in fear, imagine your parent berating you for being such a ninny; imagine flinging yourself into your father's lap, full of love, only to be told, "Stop being such a bother"; imagine the time you experienced the death of a favorite pet and felt the despair of recognizing that everything dies; and imagine the pain of being the last one chosen for a team at recess or of not having anybody to sit with in the lunch room.

Even if you don't remember any of these specific scenarios, you experienced them in some form. And they were very intense, for you felt these expectations, disappointments, and wounds more deeply and for longer periods of time when you were young. Time is different for a child. A day feels as long as a week does to an adult. A week is a lifetime. And you, like many children, probably didn't have people in your life who could help you meet and channel these feelings. So you experienced these sometimes scary and often overwhelming visitors by yourself.

On top of being afraid of the powerful feelings that moved through you, you also got the message that most of those feelings were not okay. Verbally and nonverbally, you were talked out of your emotions. The adults in your life told you: "Big girls and boys don't cry." "Sit still." "Don't make such a big deal out of it." "That is nothing to be afraid of." "Don't be so exuberant." "I'll give you something to cry about." "I am not angry!" (while screaming at the top of their lungs). Not only were you being trained to hide your feelings, but you were also being trained to distrust and dislike them.

No little body could survive the onslaught of feelings you experienced. Something had to be done to cope with them. Every time your world confused, threatened, or disappointed you, you learned to pull back, hold your breath, and tighten your body in the hopes that this would keep the painful feelings at bay. Your exuberance was confined in shallow breathing. Sadness and a deep sense of longing became hidden in your chest. Self-judgment became buried in your neck and shoulders. Fear and anger were tightly locked in your stomach. Despair, especially the despair of losing sight of your natural, free-flowing joy, was concealed deep within your belly. And underneath that despair was an empty hole that nothing could fill.

When you were young, you could control a lot of your feelings by just holding your breath, tightening your body, or getting distracted by something else. You also learned how to use your mind to make you and your life into what you thought they should be. But as we have seen, these feelings you have buried underneath a thin layer of control are *huge*. When your veneer of control wore thin, you created stronger and more elaborate systems called compulsions to keep those unmeetable feelings at bay.

After having listened to my compulsions for many years, I have learned that whenever a compulsion began in my life, *it came as a friend.* Compulsions are intricate survival systems that we create because we don't know how to be there for ourselves. They build on themselves over the years like castles with mazes of hallways, tunnels, hidden rooms, and secret dungeons. Understanding that we create our compulsions to take care of ourselves is essential in transforming our relationship to them.

Two Ways Our Compulsions Take Care of Us

Our compulsions serve two functions: the first is to keep unacceptable feelings buried deeply within so we can be numb enough to survive, and the second is to bring us comfort. In our youth most of us were not taught how to meet the unacceptable storms of rage, the dragons of fear, the rivers of sadness, and the terror of inadequacy that moved through us. Left on our own we learned how to stop these feelings by trying to be good little boys and girls. When that didn't bring us the love we needed, we learned to become very busy or to eat a whole bag of cookies or to become a really good student. As we got older many of us then got lost in the body-numbing world of alcohol and drugs.

I can vividly remember a time when I was eleven, lying in my bed late one night. After dinner I had read *Ask Andy,* a favorite column in our newspaper where you could get answers to the most obscure questions. Even though I loved it, I always felt I was too stupid to send in a question. Looking out my bedroom window, I saw Venus resting almost within the crescent of the moon.

The next morning, feeling great pleasure that I was finally smart enough to send in a question, I announced at breakfast that I was going to ask Andy why Venus and the moon were always so close together. My family let me know very derisively that this was actually a rare occurrence. I slunk away from the table like a dog that has been beaten. I can still remember that feeling in my body — the bottomless pit of self-rejection. To numb those feelings, I snuck into the kitchen after breakfast and stole some of my Dad's candy. Hiding under the table in my room, I ate the whole bag. Even though I have memories of comforting myself with food before then, this was the first memory I have of stuffing myself in an attempt to stop painful feelings.

The feelings we buried weren't always painful; we have also tried to hide from our joy. Have you ever noticed that when you are feeling really good, you find yourself drawn to your compulsion? We have been cut off from our feelings for so long that the aliveness and openness that joy brings can feel scary. And so we find ourselves wanting to hide in the familiar world of our compulsions. Whether it is fear, anxiety, irritation, anger, joy, exuberance, sadness, or despair, if we stay disconnected from our bodies and all the feelings that our bodies hold, these feelings will fuel our compulsive cycles.

Besides helping us to numb our feelings, each act of compulsion also helps us to reconnect with the deep comfort we knew when it was okay to be ourselves. This feeling that everything is all right with us and our world is a necessary component of survival. In the 1950s, Dr. Harry Harlow of the University of Wisconsin took a group of baby monkeys from their mothers at birth. They were put in cages all by themselves and then given a choice of two surrogate mothers. The first was a wire monkey that could feed them from a bottle suspended at its center. The second was a cloth monkey that, while it did not feed them, could be held close for comfort. Over and over the baby monkeys chose the comforting cloth monkey over the wire monkey that could feed them. The nourishment of comfort was more important than the nourishment of food![1]

As adults, we hold the primary source for this comfort and connection within ourselves. Of course we also need to receive it from other human beings, but if we haven't learned how to be connected with ourselves, the love and support from the outside won't penetrate our armor. Reconnecting with ourselves means living in our bodies, trusting ourselves, and being okay with ourselves, no matter what is happening. For most of us, the comfort that comes from connecting with ourselves has been taken over by the belief that we should be different from or better than what we are. This belief is based on the insidious voices in our minds that tell us we are not okay right now. And no amount of becoming better will ever quiet these voices. Just like a drop of dye in a glass of clear water, this belief can eventually permeate our entire relationship with ourselves, removing us from the essential comfort of being at ease with ourselves exactly as we are.

When we live on the endless treadmill of *I will be okay when I make myself better,* we find ourselves starving for the comfort of being at ease with ourselves. We look for the source of our comfort and meaning *out there* — in some beautiful body we haven't yet attained, in some task we haven't yet accomplished, or in some person who hasn't yet loved us the *right way.* And finding our idea of comfort missing — and even more painful, discovering it, only to watch it slip through the fingers of our control — for survival, we have to replace it with something else.

This is where compulsions enter the picture. A freshly baked cookie, a new dress, the warm glow from a glass of wine: all these relax the inner world of struggle and open the gates to the pleasure of comfort. But this comfort is short-term. If our intent in partaking of them is to relieve the pressure of not being okay with who we are, one cookie is not enough. It is like trying to scratch an itch by waving our hand in the air a few inches above our skin. So we try two cookies, and then four, and then an entire bag. Our desperate need for comfort is so great that we will keep on eating with the hope that it will bring us the peace of being comfortable in our own skins, even though it is actually doing the opposite.

I can remember another powerfully compulsive moment when I was twelve years old, right after my parents announced they were divorcing. I was sitting in a big chair at a friend's house, eating handful after handful of chocolate chips. Although I don't remember who the friend was, I vividly remember that chair and the bag of chocolate chips. It was a pivotal moment in my life, for I had finally found someone to love me. It wasn't a person; it was a bag of chocolate chips! This binge eased my agony for a few moments as the fullness in my stomach filled up the emptiness I was feeling. But this peace only lasted until I started to feel sick in mind, body, and heart.

For most of us, the wave of longing to find comfort out there has crashed against the rocky beach of despair so many times that we are finally beginning to realize that this endless craving for comfort from the outside will never satisfy us if we are not comfortable in our own skins. We are ready to see that we are really longing for a richer, deeper, more healing comfort — the comfort of loving ourselves from the inside out, connected to ourselves, to our lives, and to our inner wellsprings.

Both these ways that our compulsions have taken care of us — numbing us and offering us comfort — were at one time necessary. But now the price we pay for taking care of ourselves in this way has become too high. It is time to take care of ourselves more skillfully. As we make this shift, our compulsions can be our guide back into a deep and abiding connection with ourselves and with life. For whenever we are compulsive, all the feelings that stand in the way of this connection are close to the surface where they can be healed. The truest gift our compulsions give us is that they won't let go until they teach us how to become truly conscious and compassionate with ourselves and with others.

Core Ideas

- Compulsions are our guides back into a deep and abiding connection with ourselves, one that relaxes our minds, opens our hearts, and brings a twinkle to our eyes. To take this journey back to ourselves and into our full potential, we need to transform our relationship to our compulsions.

- Compulsions are not evidence that you are weak-willed or defective. Rather, they are powerful forces that are here to heal you to your core.

- Compulsions are a survival system created to manage all the overwhelming, disappointing, and unmeetable experiences of our lives.

- Compulsions temporarily help us to reconnect with the deep comfort we knew when it was okay to be ourselves, but this endless craving for comfort from the outside will never satisfy us if we are not comfortable in our own skin.

- These ways that our compulsions have taken care of us — numbing us and offering us comfort — were at one time necessary. But now it is time to take care of ourselves more skillfully. As we make this shift, our compulsions can be our guide back into a deep and abiding connection with ourselves and with life.

- The truest gift our compulsions give us is that they won't let go until they teach us how to become truly conscious and compassionate with ourselves and with others.

Chapter 4

LEARNING TO

Respond

Even though all our compulsions begin as friends, with specific roles to play in our lives, and even though at times we are happy to have them pay us a visit, the longer compulsions are a part of our lives, the more they become like visitors who have overstayed their welcome. This type of guest leaves dirty laundry on the floor, makes expensive calls, and eats you out of house and home. For many of us, compulsions are not just unpleasant visitors; they become mean and nasty monsters, taking over our lives and breaking our hearts.

So of course we want to get rid of them. We try everything we can think of, only to have the monster come roaring back again. It may be in a different form, but it is still compulsive behavior. We may give up drugs only to start chain-smoking. Why is this? Compulsions aren't random events that turn up just to make a mess of our lives. They are not evidence of our lack of discipline, or proof that *they* (usually our parents) screwed up, that you failed, or that whatever higher power is in charge fell asleep on the job. Instead, they are calls to awaken and will, if we learn how to listen, guide us into our *true selves,* and they will keep calling, sometimes in varied guises, until we wake up.

Odd as it may seem, compulsions, along with all the fear, self-judgment, and despair that they bring, exist to empower and heal us to our core. They come from the deepest and wisest parts of us and bring all the experiences we need to move out of the prisons of our minds. Compulsions come from our longing to trust ourselves and our lives again so we can become partners with the creative force that flows through everything.

Moving beyond Struggle

Ironically, there is practically no better teacher of how to be truly alive than our compulsions. The key to gathering all the wisdom that they bring is to transform our relationship to them. We usually live in reaction, fighting them, giving in, and then fighting again. We live in reaction to our compulsions because we hate and fear them. There is a huge difference between living in *reaction* and living in *response.* We have been trained to react. We think in terms of what should be and what shouldn't be, of what was and what will be. We push and pull, grab and resist instead of responding, instead of listening to our compulsions, learning from them, and bringing the light of our attention to what is happening right now, tapping us into the awesome power of pure curiosity.

What we resist persists. I have a very strong will. Many times I went without eating for long periods of time, only to binge uncontrollably afterward. Many times I thought I finally had this urge to overeat under control. Thank God, I was never quite able to do it. These are very powerful forces that cannot and should not be tamed. If you try to break a horse, you may be able to ride it, but the horse will have lost its spirit. If you discover how to be in true relationship with a horse, it will give you the gift of its wildness and its speed. An example of this truth is shown in the movie *Horse Whisperer,* which was based on Monty Roberts's work with gentling rather than breaking horses.

What works with horses also works with our compulsions. If we try to break them, they have a tendency to "bite us in the butt." But if we learn how to *be in relationship with them,* not only can we heal our compulsions, but we can also be healed *by* them. It was when I learned how to let go of my hatred and fear of my compulsions and became curious about what was happening inside me that I began to heal and be healed by them. Each wave of compulsion that I was able to be present for dissolved a little more of the prison of my mind and opened the door to my heart. In the beginning I was only able to be there for a moment or two, but each moment made a difference. Rather than leaving me in deep despair, my compulsive moments began to leave mercy and joy in their wake.

Even though it felt like I paid a high price for my compulsions, in the long run they have brought me much more than they have ever taken away. They didn't allow me to manage and control my way to a temporary healing that kept me separate from the lasting healing that I truly longed for. Crashing over and over against the bulkhead of my own impotence, they narrowed down my options until the only one left was to open up and engage with them. I had to allow them to bring me back to myself — not an idea of what I should be, but a true and loving connection with myself *exactly as I am.* As I was finally able to tell myself the truth of my experience and accept it — rather than being ashamed or afraid — the clouds began to part. I slowly moved from *I am not/I should be* to the wonderful and nourishing experience of *I am!* This has melted so many of what I call the "*I am not* knots" in my body, mind, and heart, helping me to joyfully open to life again.

Learning how to respond to our compulsions rather than reacting to them is a radically different experience from what we have been taught. To make this shift, it helps to look at the many gifts that we will receive as we learn how to listen to our compulsions rather than living on the pendulum of reaction. Compulsions can show us how caught we are in our heads and reveal to us the futility of domination. It is amazing how much we all believe muscling our compulsions into submission will bring us the healing that we long for, even though evidence exists that it doesn't. Remember the statistic that 95 to 98 percent of all the weight that is lost, plus some, is gained back within a year and a half. And yet diet books are perennial best-sellers. It is also true that the recidivism rate at drug rehabilitation centers and eating disorder programs is very high. And it seems that if we do control one compulsion, often another takes its place. Our compulsions are trying to teach us how to be curious. They will only let go of their grip as we learn how to respond to what is happening rather than reacting. This is a much more effective way to use our minds. Rather than constantly trying to change what is, a person who has learned how to be curious about what is happening, even for just a moment, can move through the thickest of mind states and the most closed of hearts to bring the healing of spaciousness and mercy.

As we learn how to listen to our compulsions, they will bring us back into the safety of living in our bodies, along with the pure aliveness and joy that reside there. The experience of being fully in our bodies is one of the things we are truly hungry for when we compulsively reach for a cigarette, a drink, a bite, or a credit card. Even just a little bit of dropping out of our heads and back into our bodies will put us in contact with the many gifts our bodies have to give, dramatically lessening the power of our compulsions.

Compulsions open the door back into our hearts, revealing the understanding and mercy that we are so starved for. This is one of the most important gifts that they bring, for it is in the heart that all true healing happens. Compulsions do this by revealing how closed our hearts are to many parts of ourselves. In recognizing how deep our self-judgments are, we are able to meet these disowned parts with mercy. This is the healing we long for, the healing of a loving relationship with ourselves.

Compulsions will reconnect us with the joy of making kind and wise choices. In the past, we have often made choices that were against us, causing such heartaches in our lives. As we become more curious about our compulsions, opening our hearts in the process, we make contact with an inner radar that guides us to the most kind and skillful thing to do in any given situation, especially a situation involving our compulsions. This radar contains what I call our "empowered no." This no is not against anything; rather, it is for the good of the whole. It knows when to say yes and when to say no so that we can again trust ourselves (we will discuss this at greater length later in the book).

When we overeat, overspend, or overwork, *what we are truly craving is ourselves.* We long for the joy of seeing the beauty of our own eyes and to feel the thrill of our own heartbeats. We long for the sensuous pleasure of chocolate melting in our mouths and of having that one bite be enough. We long for the freedom of a full breath rather than a puff of a cigarette. All these examples come from that wondrous relationship in which, no matter what is happening, it feels okay to be in our own skins.

Compulsions also reveal and bring clarity to all the blocks that stand in the way of knowing and living from this kind of connection with ourselves. What fuels every wave of compulsion is all the painful feelings and thoughts that we have boxed up inside us. Compulsions bring them close to the surface where they can finally be seen and then healed through understanding and mercy.

This trust of ourselves and of our lives brings us back to the truth. As Jesus once said, "You will know the truth and the truth will set you free." Most of us imagine him to be speaking about lofty ideas and concepts. Yet truth with a capital T has nothing to do with ideas *about* life. Truth is *what is* — right now. Truth is that you are sitting here reading. Truth is that you are thinking and feeling exactly what you are thinking and feeling. To let go of focusing on what you should or shouldn't be, and for just a moment to connect with the truth of *what is* taps you into your own authenticity and brings clarity, freedom, and peace.

Ultimately we have compulsions so that they can show us that we are not alone, that a power greater than us exists. This power is so awesome that it keeps the planets spinning as they do with a precision that is mind-boggling. It also orchestrates the seasons with an astonishing rhythm and even permeates every cell of our bodies. When we try to heal our compulsions solely with our minds, we are relying on a limited power. But when we learn how to use our minds to be curious, cultivating an alert appreciation for what is really going on inside of us, a wiser part of us connected to the wisdom of life begins to have a voice in the process. As we learn how to listen, answers come flowing up from deep inside of us with a clarity that is a joy to behold.

A Glimpse of What's Possible

Because we are so used to seeing our compulsions as the enemy, it may be difficult to let in the possibility not only that compulsions can be a guide back to ourselves but also that, hidden in their depths, are the treasures that we have longed for our whole lives. To get you over the hump of disbelief, in the following exercise I want to give you a glimpse of the place compulsions are trying to open you to:

Exercise

Begin to shake the hand that you are not using to hold this book. Get it going as fast as you can for a few moments. Go for the gusto so you can get your energy moving. Now close your eyes, stop shaking your hand, and bring your attention to it. Can you feel the free-flowing energy? For a few moments, enjoy this feeling of aliveness.

Now let us get a glimpse of how it feels to have energy moving throughout your whole body.

Exercise

After you read the following section, put the book down and start shaking your hand again. Let that shaking move up through your entire arm and then over to the other arm. When both your arms are involved, see where the shaking wants to go from there.

Watch for the voices in your head that want you to stay contained. The predominate voice in the beginning may be the one that comes from your *I am not/I should be* training dictating that you always have to do it "right" and look cool. Give yourself permission to move beyond that voice for these few moments and let your exuberance and your natural inclination to play come on board again. Have fun with this! Shake, rattle, and roll! (My hips love to get involved!)

Now close your eyes and stop shaking. Bring your attention into your body and enjoy the flow of energy. Let that bliss bring you fully back into your body and into yourself — not an idea of you, but the *real thing.*

We don't need to go around shaking our bodies to know the joy of true connection with ourselves and with life, the kind we all felt when we were young. All we need to do is learn how to respond to what life is bringing us, rather than living in reaction, so we can open to life again. This opening comes through a fascinated curiosity about what is happening right now and a deep willingness to meet it all with an understanding heart.

I want to share with you the first time I became open enough as an adult that the energy flowing within me could fill me with its presence. It happened early one morning right after I woke up and my mind was still very quiet. Rather than getting out of bed, I began to breathe slow and deep breaths while still snuggled under the safety of the covers.

Using my mind to connect with *what is* rather than *what was* or *what will be,* I became passionately curious about what I was experiencing right then. Immediately I noticed a tingle of aliveness throughout my whole body.

By paying attention to it, I allowed it to expand from my very core into every nook and cranny of my being. The more present I became, the more my body radiated the joy of being alive. Every once in a while the thoughts in my head would try to capture my attention, but I could easily let them go and return to being fully present with myself, with life, and with the joy of being alive. After a while my insistent mind began to take over. When I noticed that I was again paying attention only to my thoughts, I would gently bring my attention back into my body. Every time I returned, I discovered the joy had dimmed as I had held my breath and slightly tensed my body when I was caught in my head.

I began to see that my mind held on to the belief that this openness would be as bruising and as wounding as it had been when I was a child. But I am not a child anymore, and even though I had to pull back from life in order to survive when I was young, I knew as an adult that in opening to life I would thrive. With a few deep breaths and a sense of relaxing into my body, I returned over and over again to myself. I did this by pulling my attention away from the thoughts in my head and placing it back into my body and the immediacy of life. There to meet me was the free-flowing energy of being completely alive.

Oh, the thrill of that! No war was raging inside me. All expectations that I be any particular way fell away. I was back in the land of *I am!* and that was enough. In fact, it was more than enough. I was allowing myself to again be animated from my core. The joy that flooded me while I was this connected to myself nourished me deeply. This joy stayed with me as I got out of bed and opened to the day. I had had a glimpse of what was waiting for me when I learned how to open to life and live from the wellspring of energy, wisdom, and support within me.

There were still many things I had to let go of and many things I needed to relearn to know and live from my essence. I had to learn how to use my mind to engage with life rather than constantly trying to manage it (a theme I'll discuss in more detail in the next chapter). I also needed to learn how to recognize the thoughts and feelings that caused me to pull back from life. And finally, I needed to meet those thoughts and feelings with compassion and understanding.

Every step of the way, my compulsions were my guide, showing me the futility of my attempts at control and inviting me to be curious about my immediate experience. My compulsions pointed out to me the feelings I had boxed up and hidden deep in my body so that I could now work with them, touching them with my compassionate heart. Little by little, with moments of curiosity and even more wonderful moments of mercy for all my inadequacies and my fears, the wellspring within me has become more real until I can now return to it even in the middle of a busy day. I still have some boxes of feelings scattered around the house of my being that I haven't yet opened. When I become aware of those feelings, my automatic reaction is to tighten down and distract myself. But not for long! After having lived in the joy and aliveness that comes from being open to life, the loss of this kind of connection is very evident when I close up again. When I notice this, I immediately become curious and then very compassionate. As my heart opens, my body softens and my mind lets go. I can then meet these feelings and transform them back into the free-flowing energy of life.

You are reading this book because you are ready to know and live from the wellspring within you, with all the joy, nourishment, wisdom, and creativity that it holds. You are ready to stop reacting and start responding to yourself. You are ready to meet your boxed-up feelings with understanding and mercy so that you can love yourself from the inside out. And you are ready to be healed by your compulsion, which will be your guide on this journey back to yourself. Now that we can see our compulsions in a different light, not as enemies but as possible allies, we can begin to listen to them, gathering all the wisdom they are bringing us. In the next chapter we will explore how to forge this new kind of relationship.

Core Ideas

- Compulsions are not random events. They come from the deepest, wisest part of yourself, bringing all the experiences you need to unravel the web of reaction and struggle that you are caught in.

- If you listen to your compulsions, responding to them, learning from them, and bringing the light of your attention to what is happening right now, you will tap into the awesome power of pure curiosity.

- Compulsions open the door back into our hearts, revealing the understanding and mercy that we are so starved for.

- As we become more curious about our compulsions, opening our hearts in the process, we make contact with an inner radar that guides us to the most kind and skillful thing to do in any given situation, especially with our compulsions.

- Because we are so used to seeing our compulsions as the enemy, it may be difficult to let in the possibility not only that compulsions can be a guide back to ourselves but also that, hidden in their depths, are the treasures that we have longed for our whole lives.

- Compulsions come from our longing to trust ourselves and life again, to become partners with the creative force that flows through everything.

Chapter 5

MOVING FROM MANAGEMENT TO

Engagement

I f we look closely at our relationship with our compulsions, we see that we truly believe they are bad and must be fought. Because of this archaic belief, the only type of relationship we have learned is one of *management.* By the signs on fitness clubs, by the slick advertising of diet centers, and by the pages of fashion magazines, we have become brainwashed with the idea that our power lies in controlling our unwanted urges.

We try to deny, dominate, annihilate, or run from our compulsions and the feelings that fuel them, only to have both roar back with a force that astounds us. We have lived with this dynamic long enough now to see that *what we try to control controls us.* Our very resistance to our compulsions, along with our hatred and fear of all the feelings behind them, fuels what we are trying to resist.

The tricky thing is that initially managing our feelings and compulsions does appear to work, but eventually it gives diminishing returns. Remember the feeling of absolute power when you lost all that weight the first time? But the next time you couldn't stay on the diet as long or lose as much. And you stayed caught in the web of management because you believed that the only reason you had failed was that you were doing something wrong. Even when management did seem to work, if you look closely you will see that you most likely switched to another compulsion. That is why so many people gain weight after they quit smoking or smoke more after they quit drinking.

This idea that our power will come from dominating what we don't like actually causes us to lose our power in the long run. This was true in my life, and I have seen it over and over again in the lives of people who come to me for counseling. Frustrated because they see themselves as losers for having failed to control their compulsions, many of them express a heartbreaking sense of inadequacy along with the deep despair that comes from the belief that there is no way out.

Trying to manage our compulsions sends us into a downward spiral where the more we fail, the more our self-judgment turns into shame, fear turns into terror, and sadness turns into despair. Believing that our only option when these feelings are present is to eat, drink, shop, work, watch television, or turn on the computer until we're numb, we find ourselves in a vicious circle of controlling and being controlled and then back to controlling again.

One of the biggest downsides to the idea that managing our compulsions will bring us the healing that we long for is that it keeps us caught in our minds with their penchant for endless trying, doing, fixing, changing, and rearranging. This cuts us off from the very information we need in order to heal. It is like walking down a path with signs on either side that point the way. We don't notice the signs because a perpetual cloud of struggle is hanging over our heads.

As we mumble to ourselves all those have-tos and ought-tos, along with all those I can'ts and I won'ts, the cloud of confusion, self-judgment, and despair grows thicker. And yet the signs are still there. The wisdom we each carry is always speaking to us — especially during a wave of compulsion — and is waiting for us to pay attention to it. On top of that, all our mumblings come from the idea that some outer authority has the answer for us, that some diet will tell us what to eat, some book will tell us how to think, some "expert in living" will tell us how to behave.

And yet there is no better expert on our lives than us.

If we believe that something or somebody else knows what is best for us, we stop trusting ourselves. As mentioned in the last chapter, this cuts us off from our own inner radar, which knows what is appropriate for us in any given situation. And even though we have been taught to ignore it, it has never left us and is waiting for our return. Once we rediscover our inner wellspring of wisdom, we will wonder how we ever functioned without it. We will never know this wellspring as long as we stay caught in our heads, trying to manage our way to the love and freedom that we long for.

So let us now look at a new way of being with our compulsions that will take us back to a deep and abiding relationship with our inner knowing. This new kind of relationship with our compulsions is one of *engagement*, the ability to be present in a curious and open way to whatever is happening. Rather than struggling with our compulsions, engagement is about listening to and learning from them, for when we are engaged we discover that hidden within every compulsive action are the keys to our healing.

Engagement is not permission to indulge in compulsions. That would just be living in more unconsciousness. *Rather, it is the willingness to stop fighting our compulsions so we can see what is going on.* Remember those puzzles from your childhood that showed a drawing with objects hidden within it that you had to find? It may have been a knife drawn into the trunk of a tree or a cat in a cloud. You had to shift your perspective to see what was there. As we shift our perspective on our compulsions, becoming curious rather than controlling, we discover that all the clues to the healing that we long for lie in whatever experience we are having right now. Our compulsions amplify those clues so we can see them more clearly.

Engagement is neither for nor against the compulsion. *It is simply a passionate interest in what is happening and a compassionate meeting of what is there.* When we start listening curiously to what is happening either before, during, or after a wave of compulsive activity, the clouds engulfing our heads lift, and we become able to see the signs pointing the way along the path. Our attention not only fleshes out the clues, but it also highlights the hidden parts of us that are fueling the compulsion. And in adding compassion to attention, these parts are transformed in the vast region of our hearts.

Engagement is built on a foundation of respect and forgiveness. Let us look now in greater depth at the two qualities inherent in this new way of relating to our compulsions.

Cultivating Respect

Most of us have never even considered respecting our compulsions, those vast forces that come roaring up from the depths of our being. The dictionary defines *respect* as "relating to; referring to for information; take into account; to have in view." These phrases succinctly describe the type of relationship that we are cultivating. Rumi, a thirteenth-century Sufi poet, wrote about the power of this kind of respect in his poem "The Guest House":

> *This being human is a guest house. Every morning is a new arrival. A joy, a depression, a meanness, some momentary awareness comes as an unexpected visitor.*
>
> *Welcome and entertain them all. Even if they're a crowd of sorrows who violently sweep your house empty of its furniture, still, treat each guest honorably. He may be clearing you out for some new delight.*
>
> *The dark thought, the shame, the malice, meet them at the door laughing and invite them in. Be grateful for whoever comes because each has been sent as a guide from beyond!*[1]

Most of us were taught to think that if something unpleasant were happening, it was because we or somebody else had done something wrong. In this duality of right and wrong, the typical reaction to unpleasantness is to judge it as wrong and try to get rid of the unwanted guest, but this has never brought us the peace we long for.

What Rumi is alluding to is one of the great secrets of transformation. We are not given difficulties because we have screwed up or because the higher power in charge of it all has it in for us. The challenges of our lives are like weights on a weight machine. They strengthen within us the capacity to become conscious human beings. We have been given them — especially our compulsions — because the Intelligence at the heart of life longs for us to mature enough so that we can know the wellspring within us and live from its wisdom, support, and love.

It takes a keen ability to pay attention, a spacious and embracing heart, and a deep humility to consciously know and live our full potential. Just as the knights of old knew that they needed a noble adversary in order to develop their skills, we too need the great teacher of our challenges to recognize and live as ourselves.

Cultivating respect allows us to recognize that the urge to be compulsive is a very strong force, often much stronger than our attempts to control it. How many times have you tried to wrestle your compulsion to the ground, only to fail? *In the face of respect, compulsions lose their strength.* In his book *Kinship with All Life*, J. Allen Boone speaks about a woman named Grace Wiley who was a well-known snake expert. One of her core passions was to transform people's relationship with snakes. She felt that "deep within the heart of every snake is not a troublemaker but a fine gentleman who strikes only because someone has invaded his domain and cornered, frightened, or hurt him."[2]

She also loved to gentle snakes that were considered troublemakers. In a bare room with a sturdily built oblong table in the center, she would place herself at the far end of the table and become as motionless as possible. When the snake was first let out of the box, it would immediately go into defense or attack position. But to its obvious astonishment and bewilderment, there was no moving target to attack. From the moment she entered the room, she silently talked to the snake — not down to it as if it were an inferior being, but across to it with the knowing that they were each a reflection of the vast Intelligence that permeates everything. She used her favorite rule of action in all relationships: that all living things — regardless of their form, classification, or reputation — will respond to genuine interest, respect, appreciation, admiration, affection, gentleness, and courtesy.

Moving from silently communicating with the snake to actually talking to it, Grace praised it for its many excellent qualities, assuring it that it had nothing to fear. The big snake would slowly uncoil and cautiously stretch itself out along the full length of the table, finally resting its head within inches of where Grace was standing. Then she would reach out and touch its back, beginning with a soft padded stick and, when there was no resistance, with her hands. The snake would then arch its long back in catlike undulations in order to better feel the care and respect of her hands.

This is true for your compulsion as well. You have a relationship with it just as you do with friends, pets, plants, and loved ones. And it longs for Grace's rule of action — treat everything and everyone with interest, respect, appreciation, admiration, affection, gentleness, and courtesy. I know that at times you feel like it is a deadly snake, coiled in your belly and ready to strike without a moment's notice. But it only strikes because you have cornered, frightened, or hurt it through your fear and disrespect. Your compulsion can also be tamed, just as Grace tamed her snakes — not through force, but through a relationship of respect and all that it means.

Just as Grace's respect moved the snake from attack mode to calm and ease, your respect has the same effect on your compulsion. Know, however, that just like with the snake, as you begin to extend respect to these forces within you, at the beginning they may coil in anticipation of attack because that is what you have always done in the past. Slowly, as the compulsion begins to trust you, it too will uncoil under your respectful gaze, sharing with you the gifts it has been carrying.

Giving respect is not giving our compulsions free rein. Rather, it is the art of becoming a skillful host to these temporary visitors from the depths of our being. A good hostess welcomes her visitors, making them comfortable in her home. She gives them the most important gift a good hostess can give — her undivided attention. She may even extend tenderness and mercy by letting the visitors know that they are understood. But a good hostess does not let guests run amok through her house. And when it is time for the visit to come to an end, the guests are graciously bid farewell.

The first time I really learned about the power of respect was from my mentor. She had been a longtime smoker and finally realized that it was no longer appropriate. She didn't try to wrestle this compulsion to the ground. Instead she gave herself six months. Every time she lit a cigarette she would acknowledge the part of her that smoked, thanking it for all that it had done for her. She then let it know that at the end of the six months she would be saying good-bye. Two weeks before the end of the six months, she got bronchitis and was unable to smoke. She never picked up a cigarette again.

At times it can be difficult to treat these visitors with respect, for they can be very demanding and manipulative. But all we have to do is recognize that when we fight them, not only do we lose our power, but we also amplify *their* power. Remembering that they are just messengers bringing us gifts from the depths of our being helps us to stay centered in our power.

This kind of respect is not only about respecting our compulsions. *It is also about respecting ourselves for having taken on our compulsions in the first place.* What would it be like if, instead of judging yourself for being compulsive, you honored the courage of your soul to use compulsions in growing into the fullness of your potential? Feel the shift in your energy as you move from disempowerment to empowerment. Now feel the difference in your body when you shift back to the old idea that you are a failure for not having conquered your compulsions.

Rather than seeing your compulsions as proof of how weak-willed you are, understand that the more your soul longs for you to become fully yourself, the stronger will be its push to awaken you. To do this, it is always looking for ways to show you where you are caught in reaction so you can open again to the ease and peace that is right beyond the struggling mind. There is practically no better place to do this than with compulsions.

You are nothing less than a soul on a journey back to itself. As you develop a relationship of respect both for your compulsion and yourself, managing your compulsion will become less and less interesting. As you learn how to engage with it instead, you will turn a former enemy into an ally, forging a partnership that will open the door again to the joy and aliveness that is your birthright.

Learning Forgiveness

Many people misunderstand what forgiveness is really about. By forgiving you are not letting someone off the hook by giving him or her absolution. True forgiveness is something far different. It is about letting go of struggling with what has happened in our lives. It is about allowing things to be as they have been so we can move on.

If we stay in resentment or fear about something that has happened in the past, we become stuck to it like glue. One of the core wounds I received from being raped in my early twenties was my hatred of the rapist. For years, I stayed attached to the rape by getting caught in rage and bitterness. It was only when I could forgive him — *not the action but the person behind the action,* understanding that he would have to have been deeply wounded himself to violate another person in that way — that I became free from the rape and all its related trauma.

Our compulsions are also asking for our forgiveness. They are asking us to meet them in the vast regions of our hearts, understanding that they were created to help us cope. Our compulsions also long for us to ask *them* to forgive *us.* All they have gotten from us is our enmity, and they need to hear us acknowledge how nasty we have been to them. Extending forgiveness and asking for it in return removes the veil of distrust, creating an opening to a respectful and healing partnership.

As we learn how to extend forgiveness to our compulsions and receive forgiveness from them in return, we can become truly free. Let us look at how to do this so that we can then forgive ourselves to the core.

Extending Forgiveness

I began the process of forgiving my compulsion in the middle of an eating binge. Sitting on my couch with a container of ice cream in my lap and a whole row of cookies lined up along the back of the couch, I began speaking to this part of me, the one that was desperately shoving food into my face. While I don't remember exactly what I said, the following words, which I ended up writing in my first book, *Belonging to Life,* convey the feeling that I experienced in these first moments of opening the door to communication:

> *I want to get to know you. I am learning how to not hate you. In fact, I am learning how to respect you. I can see that you were birthed out of a desire to take care of me. In numbing me out, you intended that I wouldn't feel the maze of terror, self-hatred, and despair. But this never brought us the cessation of pain that we yearn for, and now you are out of control. I want to heal beyond this war that we have with each other. I want to listen to what you have to say. I want to invite you back into my heart. We have both paid a heavy price for our lack of communication.*

This little bit of connection changed my whole experience. I realized I wasn't hungry for the food. *I was hungry for the feeling of curiosity and compassion that was moving through me in that moment.* Because it was hard in the beginning to hold on to this level of compassionate attention while in the middle of an eating storm, I began to write letters to my compulsion, both to forgive it and to ask for forgiveness.

These letters kept my intent to heal and be healed in the forefront of my mind. They also allowed me to look back and see the transformation from hatred and fear to a partnership based on respect and trust. In the beginning, my letters were filled with rage and despair, with only a little of the space that comes from engagement and acceptance. At the end they were filled with gratitude, understanding, and compassion.

If you are called to write to your compulsion, a skillful way to begin is to write at the top of the page, "I am writing this letter to invite you back into my heart." This is a perfect opening line, for either it will bring up your longing to heal and words will flow from this longing or it will bring up all your rage over the abuse you have suffered at its hands. Whatever it evokes, tell your compulsion exactly how you feel. The key to writing this kind of letter is to trust exactly where you are.

Here is a paragraph from one of my letters:

I am here to invite you back into my heart. I may fear you and even hate you, but even bigger than that is my desire to heal my heart. You have caused me much pain in my life. I am beginning to realize that you are an essential part of the community of my being, and I forgive you. I forgive you for all of the embarrassment, for all of the agony, for all of the upsets you have caused. I now want to allow you back into the healing of my heart. I have grown immensely from your presence and rather than seeing you as an enemy — as a defect in my being — I realize you come from the depths of my being to awaken my heart. I forgive you.[3]

When I was forgiving my compulsion, I would always end this part by reminding it that my intention was to create a healing relationship with it. I also would remind it that sometimes I would forget this and act out of my conditioning that says I must hate and fear it. I would tell it that when I got lost again, I would make every effort to remember this commitment to partnership.

Receiving Forgiveness

For a long time, I didn't realize that forgiveness was a two-way street. I was communicating with my compulsion, but I hadn't yet opened the door to my compulsion communicating with *me*. With startling clarity, I realized one day that I was on the path of forgiving it for beating me up all those years, but I had not even contemplated opening the doors to being *forgiven by my compulsion!* I saw that every time I had put it out of my heart, it received another load of hatred and fear from me, instead of the wisdom and compassion that was necessary for it to heal. It needed for me to acknowledge that. Because I had never contemplated asking for its forgiveness, it couldn't trust my overtures. A paragraph from another letter shows the power of asking for forgiveness from our compulsions:

> *I ask you to forgive me for how much I have hated you. Rather than including you as a part of me, knowingly and unknowingly I have sent hatred and violence your way. I ask now that you forgive me for my ignorance, forgetfulness, confusion, and rage. I did not see that you were sent from my soul to awaken me. I did not see that it is in letting you back into my heart that we are both healed. I ask that you forgive me for constantly warring with you.*[4]

As I allowed myself to be forgiven by my compulsion, it began to write letters back to me! At the beginning I was a bit dismayed by the rage and hurt that it expressed, but all I had to do was remember the great violence I had sent into these wounded parts of myself, and understanding replaced my dismay. Like all beings, it just wanted to be heard. I could then make space again for it to speak its truth. I could finally hear the grief, rage, and terror that fueled my bouts of overeating. I listened to them in the way they needed to be heard when they were created in my youth.

The more I listened, the more I understood that underneath all the rage and bitterness, my compulsion carried great wisdom and had been waiting for the opportunity to share it with me. My heart began to melt, and the compulsive eater and I became friends. Because it was recognized, respected, and heard, we became partners in our healing and it didn't need to scream so loudly to get my attention.

It can be more challenging to allow your compulsions to write to you than it is to write to them. They may not be at all sure about trusting your new intention to heal. Because of this, you may not get any response at the beginning. After all, they have never had a voice. But if you are willing to keep this dialogue open, they will eventually make themselves known. Compulsions, just like people, respond to apologies and a willingness to listen.

A good way to get things flowing is to imagine what you would feel like if you were in a relationship in which someone constantly ignored you or put down everything you said. Then realize that this is how you have been with your compulsion and that it probably has something to say about that! Or, if you are beginning to listen to your compulsion, imagine what it feels like finally to be respected and heard. Then allow yourself to write down whatever thoughts and feelings come to you.

Forgiving Ourselves

If the process of forgiving your compulsion doesn't call to you right now, explore forgiving yourself. Say, "I forgive you, _____," adding your name at the end of the phrase. Just chanting this phrase can be very powerful. Either it will open your heart or it will reveal the places where your heart is still closed to you. You can amplify it by saying, "For all the mistakes in your life, for all the reactions of a closed heart, I forgive you, _____. I see now that you are an awakening being and every experience of your life was necessary on the journey. I forgive you."

Forgive the unlikable, the contracted, and even the unacceptable parts of you. Allow yourself back into your own heart. You are worthy of this kind of mercy. If your mind throws up all the reasons that you can't be forgiven, watch how unkind the mind can be, and permit this hard edge to be forgiven. Repeat these words numerous times, making them your own and allowing them to open you to a tender, caring, relationship with yourself.

In the willingness to explore forgiveness, we need to know that the roots of reaction and resentment are buried deep in all our hearts. At times, a forgiveness practice will help us to see how closed our hearts still are, and we can then explore this armoring. At other times, it will reawaken us to the spaciousness of an open heart, allowing our ancient pains to float in the healing of mercy.

As you write your forgiveness, allow not only your rage and grief but also your deep longing to heal to have a voice. Speak about the hope you have discovered as you have explored a whole new way of working with compulsions and about the awakening of your desire to discover the gifts that compulsions carry. This hope may at times turn back into distrust and the despair that nothing will ever change. Allow these feelings a voice, for they too exist as the next step in your healing. And when you are ready, share your gratitude for all that your compulsion has been trying to awaken within you. Everything responds to appreciation.

Just as in all relationships that are healing, there will be ups and downs in this process. Writing letters to your compulsion is a great way to begin. It claims your willingness to forgive and be forgiven, to heal and be healed. If it doesn't call to you to do this, trust that. The ideas that we explored in this section are powerful seeds that will grow within you in their own time and their own way. If it does call to you, keep writing. For it is a very effective way to keep the lines of communication open between you and your compulsion.

Listening to the Monster

Now that we have worked with cultivating respect for our compulsions and have practiced both giving and receiving forgiveness, we are ready to cultivate curiosity (a topic we'll explore in depth in chapter 7). After having been so thoroughly trained to believe that controlling and managing is the only way to freedom, we sometimes feel that if we become curious about our compulsions rather than always trying to control them, we will be helpless in the face of them. Nothing could be further from the truth. Our ability to listen to our compulsions exerts an influence that is a million times more powerful than any attempt at control. It allows us to see what is truly going on without the resistance that keeps compulsions going — the resistance that comes from the old style of management.

I want to share a story about the monster of compulsion living in your house. It begins with your living in reaction to this unwanted guest and gradually moves to the healing of engagement. It honors management, but shows us that it only takes us so far into the healing that we long for. This story also shows that the shift from management into engagement is gradual. What we are exploring isn't about getting rid of all our managing tools — *it is about adding curiosity to the process.* Over time managing your compulsion will become less and less interesting as engagement brings you the freedom you long for.

Imagine that you once had a friend called compulsion. This friend promised you surcease from all your pain. But, as we have all discovered, relationships can be challenging, and as this one deteriorated, this former friend turned into a monster, and you ordered him out of your house. You come home one evening after a long day at work and discover this monster still sitting in your living room.

"What are you doing here?" you ask with great indignation.

When you get no response, you become irritated, and again you order him out of the house. He doesn't move. Racing into the kitchen, you ask your family members why they let him in, and they say he just appeared. Returning to the living room, you announce that you are going to call the police, and he still does not respond.

Calling 911, you say, "There is an emergency. A monster has moved into my house, and I want you to take him away."

Kindly but firmly they tell you that this is not their job. You call social services, moving companies, and even the zoo, hoping to get rid of this unwanted guest. Nothing works. In desperation, you even toy for a while with the idea of calling in a hit man (your Uncle Joey could probably arrange it), but that idea is too abhorrent to your tastes.

Believing that you are solely responsible for your reality, you decide that the monster continues to lurk in your living room because you are not doing something right. So off to counseling you go. You describe the monster in your living room, and the counselor takes you back into your childhood, discovering a trauma there. This understanding brings deeper layers of mercy, and you let go of a big chunk of self-judgment. You drive home with a lightness in your heart and a smile on your face. With great hope you enter the living room, fully expecting the monster to be gone.

He isn't.

In your frustration, you begin to listen to what the monster seems to be saying. You become convinced that you would feel a lot better if you got lost in your compulsion, and without a second thought, you go in search of its promise of peace and comfort. The relief you get from indulging in your compulsion is temporary, leaving discomfort, judgment, and maybe even despair in its wake. So you decide you will never do that again and claim that you will now be on top of these urges from the deep. You read books that show you how to be in control, and with great perseverance you cultivate these skills. And for a while it seems that the monster of compulsion is gone, for when you go into the living room you don't see him there.

One evening, while watching television, the pile of blankets in the corner begins to move, and there, much to your dismay, is the monster. In a flash you realize that the whole time you thought you were in control again, he was taking a nap. Deep self-judgment and despair fill you, and you immediately get lost in a wave of compulsion.

After the wave moves through, you pick yourself up and say, with great determination, "This monster isn't going to get the best of me!" When you go into the living room you sit on the couch, close your eyes, and say powerful affirmations, repeating to yourself over and over again, "I am in control of myself, and this irritant is gone from my life." You feel more empowered as you repeat these words, and you know that he is evaporating right now as you speak. In a very confident move, you take a peek through your closed eyes, only to discover that he is still there!

The more you go to your compulsion for relief, the deeper your self-judgment and despair grow. For you know that you are supposed to be in control of this monster. You are certain that everybody else can do this and that you have failed only because you are weak-willed, stubborn, and rebellious. So you try program after program, each one promising that they will eliminate compulsions, thus getting rid of the monster.

The sense that he would be gone if only you could figure it all out and understand how to "do" life right begins to eat at your heart. Despair floods your being, but with great strength you affirm that you will just try harder and then it will work. One morning, after a particularly rigorous week of controlling your compulsion, along with all the counseling, affirming, and visualizing that promised to get rid of it, feelings of deep grief and rage begin to overwhelm you.

"Everybody else can get rid of their monster in their living room" (what you fail to notice is that most people can't, and if they do, another monster of compulsion usually moves in). "And if I can't get rid of mine, there must be something terribly wrong with me." You collapse on the floor in a flood of tears, self-judgment, and hopelessness.

In the middle of this storm you hear a very faint, melodious voice. "Ask me why I am here."

In shock you look up at the monster. In this whole time he had never before spoken!

"What did you say?" you ask in amazement.

"Ask me why I am here," he repeats.

"Well, I don't want to talk to you. You are the enemy. I didn't invite you into my home. You came unbidden and are deeply unwelcome," you respond. In a huff you turn your back to him.

"What have you got to lose?" he asks. "Nothing else has worked. I haven't gone away."

In your desperation you realize that this is true. Picking yourself up out of the heap of self-failure, you slowly approach him. (This whole time you've never come any closer than ten feet.) Your heart is racing wildly. "This is the enemy," you say to yourself. "What am I doing? I must be crazy. I will be overwhelmed and lost if I get any closer." But your desperation urges you on.

As you sit down on the chair across from him, the first thing you notice is that the monster has kind eyes! "Why, you have beautiful eyes," you say. "And they are even twinkling with joy and laughter. Why have I never noticed before?"

"Because you made me the enemy," he says in his melodious and healing voice. "I am not your enemy. In fact, from the depths of your being I came into your life to awaken you. I am not here to disturb you, even though I do evoke that in your mind. I am not here to harm you, even though I do bring up your fear. I am your ally, highlighting the old beliefs you have taken on about yourself that keep you separate from all that you yearn for. If you listen to that which is upsetting in your life, it will show you the way back to yourself."

In some corner of your being you know that what he is saying is true. Rather than running away, you begin to listen, and your heart begins to melt. Joy surges through your body, and you become curious about the monster rather than reacting to him.

"You truly are my friend," you say. His laughing eyes answer yes. "And you have been waiting a long time for me to pay attention and listen to what you have to say."

With a big sigh, he affirms this truth.

You realize that every time he is present, he reveals another piece of your healing. Even with this connection, at moments your fear and confusion take over. But you notice the kindness in his eyes, and again you find yourself present for this former enemy.

Something he said finally becomes clear to you. *Life is for you!* Who you really are includes both the dark and the light; the dark is being used as a tool of awakening. When you understand this, it becomes evident that your life — all of it — is trustworthy. And the deep safety you long for comes when you learn how to be present for yourself in a curious and compassionate way.

Engagement in Action

Everything we have explored so far has been about transforming our relationship with our compulsions so we can move beyond constant struggle into the ease and peace that is our birthright. An experience of mine reveals what it looks like as we transform our relationship to our compulsions from one of management to one of engagement. I share it with you to give you a glimpse of what can happen as you transform your own relation to compulsions. If you don't overeat, just substitute your own primary compulsion.

It was late and I was tired. It had been a long day with even a longer day coming. After leading a group, I had an hour's drive to my home. Into this space, like a monster from the deep, came the desire to eat. This wasn't hunger. This was a desperate craving to EAT AND EAT AND EAT AND EAT.

I hadn't had a visit from this old teacher in a long time. After a long hibernation, the part of me that wanted to eat had returned on this dark and rainy night in a powerful way.

"I want a chicken sandwich at Burger King, and I want it now!" it said. "In fact, if I don't get one, I am going to die!"

I am highly allergic to wheat, and to eat this sandwich would have devastating results. For a few moments my unconscious mind reacted, "Oh, my God, my compulsion is back!" Right after this thought came a wave of self-hatred. "What have I done wrong to have it show up again?"

But this ancient reaction lasted only a few moments, and then curiosity took over. "It feels like there is something inside me that is very vulnerable and very young and desperately needs my attention." Knowing I needed help to meet this, I asked the wellspring of wisdom inside to show me what I should do. Immediately what came to mind was the "Serenity Prayer," but in an entirely new way. Rather than asking to change anything, what came were the words, "God grant me the serenity of staying curious, the courage to be present for what is asking to be met, and the wisdom to keep my heart open."

As I drove down the road breathing long and slow breaths, and with each breath repeating these healing words, my mind calmed down. Moving out of reaction, I asked the question, "In this moment, what am I experiencing?" (In chapter 12 we will explore this question in great depth.)

I didn't ask this of my emotions, I asked it of my body. My attention settled in my body, exploring the sensations there. As I made it through the feeling of deep weariness, I found the empty hole in my stomach that fueled this rage for food. I had been so busy the previous week that I had lost a sense of my center, and this feeling of emptiness was clamoring for my attention. Instead of meeting it in the last few days and giving it the loving attention it needed, I had ignored it, and now its only option was to go back to the old pattern of trying to be filled by food.

Knowing that these feelings needed to be received, I stayed with the physical sensations, asking questions of these angry, terrified, and overwhelmed parts of me. Just in the act of responding rather than reacting, I was able to calm down the urge to eat, even though a part of me still felt that I would die if I didn't get the sandwich. Not demanding that this be any different, I spent the drive to the restaurant in openhearted, responsive communication. I knew that if I forced the compulsive eater in me at all, it would take the power and run. These feelings that fuel an eating binge are so primitive and so scared that they usually can override the best of intentions.

Close to the freeway exit where the restaurant was, I felt we had progressed far enough that I reminded myself how ill I would feel if I ate wheat. Making space and truly respecting and listening to these feelings created the possibility of compromise. Rather than a sandwich, which would make me sick, I suggested a big bowl of quinoa (a grain that my body loves) along with lots of toasted sesame oil — all to come when I got home. The desperate desire for the sandwich faded away, and I drove by the exit. I then had a few moments of panic as the eater raged. "You fool!" it said. "You missed the chance to eat what you really wanted." I felt a surge of anger at myself for not having followed my compulsion. But then curiosity kicked in again, and rather than following this thought, I could see what the eater was doing.

This ancient and lumbering beast truly felt that the only avenue of comfort was something that would bring devastation in its wake. I reminded it of the joy that comes from making a kind choice and how much better I would feel tomorrow after eating something healthy.

When I got home, I crawled into bed with my bowl of quinoa (with extra oil!) and turned on my heating pad. I knew that in responding to what was going on rather than reacting to it, I had taken another step beyond struggle, another step back into myself and all the joy, aliveness, wisdom, and support that reside there.

It is safe to be curious about what we are experiencing when we are compulsive. It is not only safe — it is the path to healing. We start this process of engaging with our compulsions gradually. We don't let go of all our old methods of control in the beginning. That would be like throwing someone in the middle of the ocean to teach her how to swim! Instead we just go sit by the ocean and contemplate the possibility of being curious about our compulsions rather than always reacting, opening to the possibility that maybe we don't need to keep fighting and struggling forever. Then we put one toe in the water, feeling for a moment the truth that our compulsions come from the depth of our being to heal us, not to destroy us. As we become more curious, we learn how to engage with them rather than constantly trying to manage them, and one day we find ourselves floating in the warm ocean of our own true nature. With deep gratitude we thank our compulsions for taking us there.

You too can know this healing relationship. In the next chapters we will explore the four skills at the core of engagement. Each of these skills will help you immensely on your path toward healing and being healed by your compulsion.

Core Ideas

- Compulsions do not show up because you are doing something wrong.

- Initially, managing your feelings and compulsions does appear to work, but eventually it gives diminishing returns. If you manage to control one compulsion, another one usually pops up to take its place.

- The key to gathering all the wisdom that compulsions bring is to transform your relationship with them from one of management to engagement.

- Engagement is about listening to and learning from our compulsions, for when we are engaged we trust that hidden within every compulsive action are the keys to our healing.

- Engagement isn't about *getting rid of* all your management tools. It is about *adding* curiosity and compassion to the process.

- Engagement is built on a foundation of respect and forgiveness. In the face of respect, compulsions lose their power over you and instead become allies, sharing with you the gifts they have been carrying.

- True forgiveness is about letting go of struggling with *what is*. As we learn how to extend forgiveness to our compulsions and receive forgiveness from them in return, we can become truly free.

- It is safe to be curious about what we are experiencing when we are compulsive. It is not only safe — it is the path to our healing.

PART THREE

FOUR BASIC SKILLS FOR WORKING WITH

Compulsions

Chapter 6

SOME FUNDAMENTALS FOR LEARNING THE
Skills

As we realize that our customary ways of working with the challenges in our lives — compulsions, a difficult boss, even international conflicts — do not bring the healing we long for, we become more open to exploring new ways of working with, learning from, and eventually being healed by the very things we formerly resisted and tried to control.

In this book, we are using our compulsions to explore a different and very healing way to work with the challenges of our lives. Even to contemplate changing our relationship to compulsions — our great teachers — from trying to manage and dominate them to becoming empowered through engaging with them, is a significant step. It opens up the possibility of listening to and learning from our experiences rather than always trying to fight or flee.

To learn how to listen to and gather all the wisdom that compulsions are bringing us, we can cultivate some basic skills. These are different from the skills of management we have relied on to maneuver through our lives — they are the skills of engagement. The following analogy will help you see the difference between our old controlling ways and the new skills we will be exploring. It also shows us where these new skills are trying to take us.

I would like you to imagine a wonderful field, a vast field that makes you feel light and joyous even to contemplate it. It may be a beautiful mountain meadow surrounded by snowcapped peaks and sprinkled with wildflowers. My own field is full of golden rolling hills that are dotted with spreading oak trees and crisscrossed with beautiful streams. The field you picture represents the depth and breadth of who you truly are. Even though you may have no memories of it, you lived in this field when you were very young, and it is still with you. It is the essence of *being* that is always with you, no matter where you are, no matter what is happening in your life.

Now imagine in the middle of your field a stand of corn that represents the human mind. When you were young, you played in this stand of corn, but you always came back to the field of *being*. But the older you became the more trails and pathways you made into your mind. Over time, this cornfield became a corn maze that eventually became your entire world, cutting you off from any contact with the field.

Just imagine the limited view you would have inside the maze. Can you see the field? No. Can you rest in the field and revel in its beauty? No. Can you feel the love in the field that shows up as the beauty of flowers, the music of water, the vastness of the sky? Again, no. To have our entire world be the corn maze of our minds cuts us off from the joy of living in the field of our being and of our partnership with the vast Intelligence that orchestrates life.

Still, we can experience and accomplish many wonderful things inside the maze. In fact, we can even make designer mazes! But we are in contact with such a small part of who we really are. And if we could put a microphone into most people's mazes, we would hear them living in a world of endless trying. Sometimes this process is very subtle, but it is almost always painful. Most of us feel responsible for whatever has come into our lives and responsible for getting our lives "together." Imagine going around and around in the maze, coming to numerous dead-ends, feeling the frustration and eventual despair that come from not being able to "do" life right. If we are lucky our endless trying will become uncomfortable enough that we begin to ask ourselves, "Is there another way to the peace that I long for?"

This is a powerful moment in our journey back to ourselves. It is the moment when we let go of the idea that we are failures because we haven't been able to control ourselves or to create the life we wanted. Instead we become willing to listen to and learn from the experiences that life gives us. This is like somebody arriving with a hot air balloon and sending down a ladder that you then climb up. From this vantage point it becomes easy to see that you are caught in the maze of your mind and that it is only a small part of who you truly are. It is also easy to see that there are pathways out of the maze.

You can also see that you have been using the skills of the maze to try to get out of the maze — the skills of fixing, trying, comparing, expecting, and judging. And it is now clear that these skills just create *more* maze! In contrast, the skills from the field are entirely different. They aren't about trying to change, fix, or get rid of anything. They aren't for or against anything. They are all about being present for *what is*, dissolving the maze through the light of our compassionate attention. This is the art of engagement. And its power is beyond anything that we have ever tried before.

Engagement is about stilling our internal struggle. We also become willing, maybe for just a moment, to let go of the illusion that we have to do it all by ourselves, and we ask for help. Having lived in the field for many years now, I can speak a truth that is at the core of existence: the field waits for us to ask for help. "But," you say, "I have asked for help so many times." The kind of asking that the field waits for is probably different from anything you have tried before. It isn't asking for the pains of our lives to be lifted. It isn't even asking for all the good stuff. It is the kind of asking that says, "Show me how to open to the life that has been given to me." This kind of asking finally helps you to understand that life is smarter than you and is giving you the exact set of experiences you need to recognize the maze and become free of it. This kind of asking also knows that ultimately you are not going to get yourself to the field on your own. The Intelligence at the heart of life will bring you there. (In part 4 we will explore asking this kind of question in depth.)

As soon as you ask for help in this way, the field begins to celebrate. It has watched you for years, caught in the endless pathways of the maze, and has been waiting for this moment. And it marshals every resource to show you how to become free of the maze. For a while it may not seem like much is happening, but it is, underneath your everyday awareness. Slowly, through the help of your compulsions, your maze will dissolve and you will again know and live from the field of your *being*.

Four Simple Concepts

Before we explore the skills of the field, we can cultivate four fundamental concepts to help us make the best use of our new skills. These concepts help to lessen the power of the corn maze to seduce us into the old world of struggling with our compulsions.

Permission to Be Conscious

Letting go of managing our compulsions is not giving our compulsions permission to run amok. Instead, it is *giving ourselves permission to be conscious*. It is the art of slowly letting go of control so that we can bring curiosity to the process. It is also about not fanning the flame of compulsions through control, so that our lives can come back into balance.

In the beginning when you let go of your tight grip on control, your compulsion may go a little crazy for a while. But this wave of reaction will calm down as you explore the art of engagement. For underneath this rebellion, your compulsion has a deep longing to be included in the healing consciousness of a curious mind and an understanding heart. It also is a little tired and overwhelmed, having borne the full responsibility of taking care of your feelings for all these years. The opposite of control is not being "out of control." Rather, it is about bringing curiosity, clarity, and compassion to whatever we are experiencing.

Patience

We won't change our old pattern of managing our compulsions overnight. We all have deeply bought into the belief that we are compulsive because we are doing something wrong and that the only way to get back into balance is to stop the behavior. On the road back to ourselves, we will get lost in this old belief over and over again. But as we cultivate these new skills, not only will we be able to work with the power of curiosity, we will also see that in trying to control our compulsions we end up being controlled.

We have also been trained to expect immediate results. "Lose ten pounds in ten days," says the tabloid headline, and we buy into it hook, line, and sinker. *What we are exploring here is not a quick fix but it is the pathway to freedom.* One of the greatest gifts you can give yourself is patience. It has taken you a long time to get thoroughly lost in the maze of reaction and struggle, trying to fight your way to freedom. It will take some time to find your way out again. You can try the quick fixes again (and you probably will), only to find yourself more deeply caught in the maze of disempowerment, self-judgment, and despair. Or you can walk, step-by-step, out of the maze.

In cultivating patience, we need to understand that compulsions come in waves. I didn't understand this for a long time. That is probably because between the ages of eleven and thirty-three, I was caught in one continuous wave of compulsion. Either I was lost in one of my many compulsions — eating, drinking, taking pills, or getting very, very busy — or I was trying to dominate them, lost in deep self-judgment and despair over my failure to control them.

Slowly, as I let go of my addiction to trying to control my compulsions, it began to dawn on me that I wasn't hungry for all those cookies, candies, chips, and ice cream that I would gorge on. What I was hungry for was my own attention! As I learned how to be present for myself, eating unskillfully became less and less interesting. In those years of slowly, step-by-step coming back to myself, a pattern began to develop. Rather than being buffeted about by continuous waves of compulsion — in which I was either trying to control them or being controlled by them — I began to experience longer periods of time between the waves. This wasn't always true, especially when I became too tired and stressed (I was raising two children by myself), but over time this new pattern became evident. Not only that, but my compulsions taught me to be passionately curious about what was going on in my inner world. So I started to learn from the waves of compulsion when they came. The more curious I became, the shorter the waves were.

Now there are very long times between waves of compulsion, and they are more like little ripples when they do come. I am connected enough to myself that I have become very savvy. I can recognize the times when I could become vulnerable to compulsions again, and most of the time I can make kind and skillful choices. There are still times where the little ripples of compulsion in my life turn into a small wave. If I can't negotiate or compromise with these sometimes primal urges, I then give myself permission to be compulsive. *But this isn't permission just to indulge. It is nonresistance, coupled with curiosity.* Every time I do this, I gain another piece of wisdom from my compulsions. In fact, the waves are so far apart now that I actually trust them when they come.

So give yourself time. You don't have to do this all at once. You just have to deal with what is going on right now. Know that there may be a phase in the beginning when it doesn't seem like much is happening and you may feel discouraged. Because you cannot yet see the benevolence of this journey back to yourself, it is easy to mistrust it. But over and over I have seen people who, measuring their progress by the old standard, don't feel like they are making very much headway. And then, just like the sun breaking through the clouds on a winter day, they turn a corner, and their whole relationship with their compulsions and with themselves changes. It is wonderful to share in their joy during these times of inner transformation.

Discovering Your Truth

I also want you to understand that ultimately you don't have to *do* anything with what is being offered in this book. The most important thing is just to read it. Each chapter will contain ideas and techniques that you can incorporate into your daily life, but this is not a *have-to* book. The core ideas of each chapter are more like precious seeds that will be planted within you as you read them and *will grow inside you in their own time and their own way.* What they grow into will be *your truth —* not somebody else's idea of how you should heal, but your unique pathway back to yourself. For nobody knows how to heal you better than *you.*

As you read this book, claim what is true for you and leave the rest. From these pieces of your own truth you will find your way back to yourself and back to life. This is the new way of healing — from the inside out. The old way was from the top down: your head takes on somebody else's idea of how you should be, and then you try to legislate it into your life. We have all done this enough to see that it has never brought us the healing that we long for. *When you heal from the inside out, you listen deeply to yourself, trusting your own unique timetable for healing.*

Listen carefully as you read the following four chapters, each of which will cover a different skill. Some skills will call to you more than others. Those will bring hope into your heart and an open breath to your body. Play with those skills. Don't make any of them into something you have to do. Instead, bring them into your life as gifts you are willing to give to yourself.

Honoring Resistance and Rebellion

Trying to heal compulsions through managing them is like standing knee-deep in a mountain stream, desperately trying to catch a fish with your hands. All it does is get you wet and frustrated. Now that you are reading this book, you are finally realizing that you don't need to dominate your compulsion. You can engage with it instead, sitting on the banks of the river of your life, putting your fishing pole of curiosity and compassion into the river of your experience in order to "catch" what wants to be healed.

Healing and being healed by our compulsions is a little like fly-fishing. As you stand by the stream of your life, casting your line of curiosity into the river of your experience, your compulsion will begin to nibble at your line and will eventually catch hold. To land the fish of your compulsion, you need to *honor your resistance and rebellion.* If you have ever been fishing, or even seen somebody else fishing, you see that as the fisherman reels the fish in sometimes the fish fights so hard that it almost slips away. What the fisherman does in that moment is to let the line out to give the fish room to move.

The same principle is true in healing our compulsions. There are times in this journey back to ourselves when the last thing we want to do is pay attention, and any attempt to be curious and merciful is met with resistance. These are the times when our attention is too scattered and our heart too closed. It is okay to honor the resistance and to turn away.

I have gone so deeply into my healing because I trust my resistance. In those times when I could feel that my resistance was stronger than my ability to stay curious, I learned how to trust it. It was telling me that I hadn't yet built the capacity to open to whatever I was experiencing. I would then back off either into the mercy of my heart or into the wonderful world of distraction. If you have ever been around a young child, you know the amazing power of distraction. A child might throw a temper tantrum because he can't have a third Popsicle in a row. You hand him a magnifying glass instead, showing him the amazing world of a magnified rock, and the tantrum transforms into curiosity!

As adults, we also need to cultivate the skill of constructive distraction, because the feelings we will uncover as we unravel our compulsions are very young, very vulnerable, and very scared. There are times to meet the feelings, and there are times not to. Distraction is the art of doing something just to have fun, forgetting for a while all this stuff about growing and healing. It is also the art of numbing out in the kindest way we can discover — renting three videos, turning off the phone and reading an entire novel in a day, or going to visit an entertaining friend.

To trust resistance is to trust your own process, remembering that a ripening is taking place within you. In your ripening, there are times to be curious about what is going on, there are times to turn away, and there are times when it is important to distract yourself. To trust resistance allows us to stay in the healing journey for the long haul. The biggest downside to not honoring our resistance is that it will inevitably turn into rebellion. Through fighting rather than listening, we find ourselves creating a monster within us that says no when we say yes, and yes when we say no. We've all been there. Every good intention flies out the window, and we find our compulsions vehemently defending their right to direct our actions.

We also know how seductive this rebellion can be. I can remember a time when I was white-knuckling myself into submission shortly after I was told that I couldn't eat wheat any more. I could feel a volcano building inside me, but at that point the only skill I possessed was trying to dominate my urge to eat wheat. In the middle of this, I woke up one day with the absolutely logical idea that I may not be able to eat wheat, but of course that didn't mean *whole* wheat! Well, anybody in his or her right mind knows that wheat is wheat, but I was so deep in rebellion mode that I could convince myself of anything.

This rebellion doesn't just show up in regard to compulsions. Think about how many times you have committed to a kind and skillful choice, only to find yourself doing the opposite. Why is this? It is because we have been taught to be soldiers. A soldier is trained to annihilate his enemy, and that is exactly what we do with our compulsions. In trying to annihilate them, we create an opposing, and usually very rebellious, force that can eventually take over our lives.

To recognize the way conquering something only creates resistance, all we have to do is look at the ebb and flow of war. In country after country, when a stronger force comes in and tries to take over, there is a natural urge to resist. And that resistance can be very, very tenacious. Even if a country has been seemingly conquered, the urge to rebel usually goes underground and can continue to foster revolution right under the conqueror's nose. Iraq, Afghanistan, Bosnia, and Northern Ireland are good examples of the way in which resistance is handed down through generations.

As I look back on my journey, I can see how I lost the ability to make kind and skillful choices. Forgetting how to listen to myself, I read every book, I tried every program, and I followed every idea I could find out there that promised me relief from my compulsion. I approached every one like a great soldier. I could muscle my compulsion underground and sometimes even control my urge to overeat, losing as many as ten pounds in a week. But it never lasted, and over time I had less and less success.

The rebellious one inside me gained more and more power with every attempt to annihilate my compulsion. The overeater within would hear the voice of the soldier: "You can't do this. You have to do this. You should have done that," and rebellion would dig in its heels with a vengeance that none of my efforts at controlling could equal. Because I was bullying and belittling rather than listening, my rebellious part became shrewd, devious, and all-encompassing. It eventually became stronger than any of my attempts to control it. I thought this was because I was just an undisciplined human being. I didn't recognize that my rebellion was being created and fed by my resistance to my compulsions.

Having not been taught any other way, I got lost in an endless cycle of conquering only to be conquered. The part of me that knew the right thing to do was continually being overridden by this intractably rebellious "no." The dentist told me to floss my teeth, and even though my gums were bleeding and there was floss by my bed, in my car, in my purse, and in the bathroom, I resisted. I was also a sporadic meditator for years, even though I had seen the tremendous benefits of a regular meditation practice. And though my back hurt so much at times that I could hardly sit, I would begin an exercise program only to give up after the first few days. I now enjoy doing all these things daily. On top of that, I eat wisely and experience the joy of bringing vitality and health to my whole body.

How have I come to know this healing place after living in endless war for decades? I discovered it by learning how to be a warrior rather than a soldier. A warrior operates from his or her sense of integrity and honor. Rather than seeing enemies, warriors realize that to reach their true potential, they need noble adversaries. Their intent isn't to destroy. Rather, it is to engage with their adversary so that they come away with more of themselves. In this engagement, they are very observant, knowing that their true power comes from respecting and getting to know their adversary — watching and learning how she operates. Fighting is the last option for a warrior, who understands that fighting is a crude and messy way to triumph and that such triumphs will be only temporary. *Compulsions won't let us go until they teach us how to be true warriors.* This is why they are a call from the depths of our being to awaken.

As you prepare to cultivate new skills, keep in mind that you can't make this journey back to yourself go any faster than it needs to go. Nor can you slow it down. You are part of a process that is much wiser than you. Know also that you may try to use these skills simply to stop your compulsion. But every time you let go of the desire to be somewhere other than where you are and are present for yourself instead — whether it is a wave of compulsion, a busy day, or just taking a shower — you take another step into your healing. Those moments when you are curious about what is happening rather than living in reaction are powerful beyond your wildest dreams. Even though they may feel like just a drop in a bucket, one day you will discover that your bucket is filled to the brim and your life is spilling over with the joy of being fully connected to you.

In the next chapters we will explore the four skills for healing and being healed by our compulsions — Cultivating Curiosity in chapter 7, Loving Ourselves from the Inside Out in chapter 8, Opening to Our Breath in chapter 9, and Coming Home to Ourselves in chapter 10. Now that you know that it is possible to trust yourself and your life again, let us turn to these skills.

Core Ideas

- The basic skills for working with compulsions are not about *doing* something to stop them — that only fuels more compulsions. They aren't about trying to change, fix, or get rid of anything. They aren't for or against anything. They are all about being present for *what is,* dissolving the maze of the reactive mind through the light of our compassionate attention.

- Letting go of controlling compulsions is not the same as giving yourself permission to be compulsive. Rather, it is an invitation to be conscious.

- Patience is a vital ingredient on the journey back to yourself. It took a long time to weave the web of compulsion, and it will take a while to unravel it.

- You don't have to do this all at once. The next step in your healing lies in what is happening right now.

- The ideas in each chapter of this book are like precious seeds that will grow in their own time. They allow you to heal from the inside out, learning how to listen deeply to yourself, trusting your own unique timetable for healing.

- To trust resistance is to trust your own process, remembering that a ripening is taking place inside you.

- A warrior operates from his or her sense of integrity and honor. Rather than seeing enemies, warriors realize that to reach their true potential, they need noble adversaries. Their intent isn't to destroy. Rather, it is to engage with their adversary so that they come away with more of themselves. Compulsions won't let us go until they teach us how to be true warriors.

Chapter 7

SKILL ONE:
CULTIVATING

Curiosity

I f you watch young children, you will see that they are passionately present. Rather than living in ideas *about* life, they are truly here. Let us glimpse what that is like through the following exercise:

Exercise

After you read this paragraph, lift your eyes from the book, and without changing anything, notice what is. See where you are. Don't just look, see! Be present. Now shift your focus to one thing that is close by — your hand, a lamp, or a pet — and see it as if you have just arrived from another planet. Be fascinated. Finally, shift your focus to the rising and falling of your breath. For just a few moments, recognize and feel it. Be curious about the wonderful gift of breath. When you are ready, bring your attention back to the page.

If you are like most people, you were probably only able to be present for a moment or two before ideas *about life* took over again. But even a moment or two can show us that there is a big difference between being lost in ideas and being fully present. Cultivating Curiosity, our first skill, is an excellent way to cut through the clouds in your mind. You could say that curiosity is the zoom lens of your mind allowing you to let go of the wide-angle view that includes past and future so that you can be present with what is right now. Most of us have left curiosity far behind in our childhoods. It has been captured by a constant stream of thought. From the moment we open our eyes in the morning until after we close them at night, our attention attaches itself to all the thoughts in our heads and then goes wherever they do. It is said that we can have as many as 65,000 thoughts a day, and 95 percent of them are repeats from the day before! You'd think we'd get bored, but we don't. These thoughts build a fascinating story in our heads that is full of all sorts of themes, the core one being that if you make yourself into the right kind of person and your life into the right kind of life, you will know the peace that you long for. None of this story is new. This endless maze of trying, of thoughts chasing themselves through our heads like a dog chasing its tail, is often so subtle we hardly notice it except as a faint undercurrent of unease. When it does explode into the big struggles of our lives — and this happens to all of us — we can begin to see how desperately this story in our heads tries to control our life. We can also see how much it loves to judge how we are doing and how easily it makes problems out of the smallest things. And yet right underneath our busy, busy minds lies another world of pure connection with life that brings us ease, joy, and love.

If you are like most people, perhaps you are asking, "Yes, but how do I get rid of this struggling mind so I can know the peace that is waiting for me?" The answer we usually get is that we must do away with struggle. But doing that would just be more struggle! One of the core skills for helping us move out of the attic of the struggling mind and back into the peace and joy of the house of our *being* is to cultivate curiosity. Why curiosity? Because it is a neutral force that has nothing to do with struggle. It doesn't want or need to change anything. Curiosity simply wants to see what is, for it comes from the wisest part of us that knows that no matter what is happening in our lives, we'll be okay.

Curiosity is focused attention. It is neither for nor against whatever it focuses on. It is simply interested in what is happening right now, whether it is a feeling inside us, the beauty of a sunset, or the tears of a loved one. Because it doesn't want to change anything, it takes us out of our minds and taps us into the present moment and our wellspring of deep knowing that we can access there. Its beauty lies in its simplicity, yet it is powerful beyond our ordinary comprehension.

As young children, we were naturally curious about and engaged with whatever was happening. But as we grew up, we were taught that our power came from fixing, changing, dominating, and controlling our lives, especially our compulsions. This has kept us on an endless pendulum of controlling, only to be controlled. The power of our attention has become like weak winter sunlight. When we relearn how to be curious about what is happening, it is like putting the weak sunlight through a magnifying glass. That light can then literally start a fire! It is the same with our focused attention: it can transform whatever it rests on.

The Great Gifts of Curiosity

The skill of cultivating curiosity comes first, because without it we would still be lost in the corn maze. It invites us *to stop striving for results and to start meeting things as they are.* There is a direct relationship between the quality of our curiosity and the depth of our healing. Very simply, curiosity cuts through the maze and provides the nourishment and the information we need to return to the field of *being.* Cultivating curiosity brings us five gifts that will help us to heal and be healed by our compulsions. Let us explore each of these in depth.

Contact with Life

In our homesickness for ourselves we become vulnerable to compulsions. They promise us the sun, the moon, and the stars and instead leave frustration, self-judgment, and despair in their wake. The reason that bending to our compulsions never truly satisfies us is that they cannot give us what we desire — the contentment, ease, and joy that come from being fully connected to ourselves and to life. I invite you to explore the present moment again, taking this experience a bit deeper.

Exercise

Put down the book and explore with deep curiosity exactly where you are. All the millions of moments of your life have led you to this day, to this place you are sitting in, and to this moment. Everything, absolutely everything, about this moment is brand new. You will never, ever again experience life as it is right now. Open yourself to it!

Notice the quality of the light. Hear the symphony of sounds all around you. Feel the river of sensations that is your body. In this doorway between past and future, what is here to meet you is ease, contentment, and, even though you may not recognize it yet, joy. Whenever your mind takes over, for these few moments, let it go. Explore life as it is right now as deeply as you can, and when you are ready, pick up the book and begin reading again.

You have just experienced moments of pure curiosity. It probably wasn't continuous. You had moments when you were using your attention to be fully present for life. You also had moments when you crawled back into the attic of your mind with ideas such as "This is boring" or "I am not doing this right" or "I need to take a painting class so that I can paint the light." Off you went into ideas about life, leaving the present behind. Every time you return to the attic of your mind, the living moment of your life goes by untouched and unused. But the house of your being is always waiting for you, right below the endless stories in your head.

Cultivating curiosity moves us beyond ideas about life into fully engaging with the present moment and all the wonder, joy, and support that reside there. It gives us what we have been looking for through our compulsions, a full connection with life again, no matter where we are, no matter what is happening. Joseph Campbell, author of *The Power of Myth*, understood this truth when he said, "People say what we're all seeking is a meaning for life. I don't think that's what we're really seeking. I think that what we're seeking is an experience of being alive so that our life experiences on the purely physical plane will have resonance within our innermost being and reality, so that we actually feel the rapture of being alive."[1]

When we are purely present with something, whether it is the beauty of a flower or the grief welling up inside us, we tap into the rapture of being alive. The alertness of curiosity transforms the smallest things and the most ordinary moments. At the same time, it takes the charge out of the deepest pains, allowing them the space to flow through us as they did when we were young. Because curiosity allows things to be, we can finally see the absolute perfection of this moment.

Just a little bit of paying pure attention to our present experience — the smell of a newly mown lawn, the taste of a ripe, succulent strawberry, the symphony of songbirds — will tell us in no uncertain terms that most of us are starving for pure experience. When was the last time you walked barefoot in soft, velvety grass, lay on the Earth and watched the clouds race by, or swung on a swing in pure joy? When was the last time you really tasted your food or truly saw your loved one's face? As adults, we don't see things as much as we *think* about what we see. We don't taste things as much as we shovel and swallow. And we are usually so lost in our minds that we rarely hear the astounding symphony of life. This brings us a life of isolation, with us starving for a deep connection with life, much as a person imprisoned in a dungeon hungers for the light.

This starvation mode makes us vulnerable to the cravings of our compulsions and their chant of "more, more, more." One bite of a delicious piece of cake is not enough, so we take bite after bite, hoping to make immediate contact with the wonders of taste, only to have the compulsion take us over as we shove more and more into our emptiness. This is not just true for overeating. All compulsions are an attempt to fill our inner emptiness so that we may know a few moments of peace.

The first time I fully understood the difference between being caught in my mind and being truly present for life was when I was attending my first meditation retreat, which involved ten days of silence in the wilds of Canada. It felt like I was being asked to do the Iron Man Triathlon without having trained! It also rained for nine out of the ten days, and the only heat was in the meditation hall. Boy, did my mind struggle! If I hadn't ridden with another woman, I would have left.

On the eighth day, I was doing walking meditation in a park next door to the retreat center. In pouring rain, with a garbage bag tied around my waist so I could maintain some semblance of dryness, I was walking back and forth while my mind was having a meltdown. "I don't know how to do this. I can't do it right. I never do anything right. There is no way out of the endless struggle of my life." I was crying, and it felt like more tears were pouring out of me than there were raindrops falling from the sky.

Then, as I walked under a tree, a huge drop of water was dislodged from the limb above my head. It fell into a puddle beside my foot, making a sound that was different from the sound of the rain. As I watched the beauty of the ripples dancing across the puddle, I was moved by wonder. One moment I was lost in my struggling mind, and the next moment I was fully there. My heart and my senses opened in delight. The rain, rather than being the enemy, became some of the most beautiful music I had ever heard. The formerly dark and brooding forest became a land bursting with life.

Just a little bit of curiosity about what was happening *right now* brought me out of the narrow confines of my mind, allowing me to make immediate contact with life. I rested in that deep peace for at least an hour before my struggles took over again. I now knew something besides the endless struggle I had been lost in for decades.

The magic and the mystery of those moments were a keyhole glimpse into the world of aliveness and joy that we all long for and that is our birthright. It was enough to keep me going for years, as slowly I was able to see all the parts of my ancient belief systems that fueled my compulsions and kept me almost completely cut off from life. Every step of the way, curiosity gave me the nourishment I had formerly been trying to get through my compulsions. Each moment that I was curious transformed my life from a B-grade black-and-white movie into a surround-sound, Technicolor wonder. Essentially, the more present I was, the less interesting my compulsions became.

Connection with Ourselves

As I've stated many times already, we are all deeply homesick for ourselves. We wake up to ourselves every morning and go to sleep with ourselves every night. Yet most of the time we don't know how to be *present for* ourselves. Stephen Levine once said that in all our searching for love "out there," what we truly long for is to hear "I love you" from ourselves. We can't know this love if we can't be present for ourselves.

Curiosity can cut through the maze of our minds so that we notice ourselves again. When I was six, I used to walk to school across a golf course with many maple trees, and I remember the joy of being in my body and of playing with the leaves. I then became so lost in the corn maze of my mind that I didn't even notice fall leaves again until I was twenty-eight. I can vividly remember the first fall I was awake again to the stunning colors of the leaves. I used to search out all my favorite pockets of color around town, for every time I was moved by the stupendous beauty of color, I would feel alive again.

But I hadn't yet learned how to be present for myself. It was many years before I could see through my self-hatred and despair so that I could feel my body again. In fact, when I first started meditating, paying attention to my breath felt too intimate. So I listened to sounds or kept my eyes open and watched the light. But slowly I was able at least to notice my body, and then eventually to inhabit it, and then finally, wonder of wonders, to come inside myself and find all the treasures hidden there.

As I came back to myself, over and over I would get lost in reaction and resistance. And over and over, I would remind myself simply to be curious about what was going on right now. Little by little, curiosity brought me back into a deep and abiding relationship with myself.

Information

Life is not a random series of events, disconnected from one another. Rather, it is a highly intelligent and intentional process in which every experience speaks to us, giving us the clues to our healing. This is especially true with our compulsions. They are not just uncontrollable urges that are out to get us — they are messages from the depths of our being, and they are loaded with information. Rather than being lost in them, if we learn how to be curious about what is going on before, during, or after a wave of compulsion, we can gain valuable insights that will bring us the healing we so desire and deserve.

Krishnamurti, the author of many books about being in the present moment, wrote about the power of observation (his name for curiosity). He was writing about fear, but we could easily replace that word with *compulsions,* and it would speak directly to what we are exploring here: "It is not that you must be free from fear. The moment you try to free yourself from fear, you create resistance against fear. Resistance in any form does not end fear. What is needed, rather than running away or controlling or suppressing or any other resistance, is understanding fear; that means watch it, learn about it, come directly into contact with it. We are to learn *about* fear, not how to escape from it, not how to resist it."[2]

As we learn how to be curious, we can begin to find our way out of the maze of compulsions — for the clues are always there. As you begin to watch, the first thing to notice is that usually *compulsions come in waves.* In other words, you are not always compulsive! It is easy to miss this fact because you are so thrilled when a compulsion is gone that you try to tell yourself it will never, ever return. When you do this, you are no longer alert to the onset of a new wave.

When you are alert, you can then see that each wave of compulsion has three distinct phases: the buildup, the middle, where we become lost in the wave, and the aftermath. Rather than being helplessly caught up in each phase of the wave, as you learn how to pay attention, you will gain information that will allow you to make clear and kind choices, even in the face of a strong wave of compulsion. I want to give you a glimpse of the healing that curiosity can bring during each of these phases. Later, in chapter 15, we will explore in depth what we can do during each phase of a compulsive wave. And even if your compulsion doesn't seem to come in waves, you can use the skills any time you become aware of being compulsive.

As the wave begins to build. When we have learned to respect and listen to our compulsion, we become attuned to its rhythms and can feel a wave just as it is beginning. This is when our compulsion promises nothing but bliss, and we follow this idea like the children in the fairy-tale followed the Pied Piper. This is the easiest time to become free from compulsion's spell, by learning the art of making wise and kind choices. At times we will be able to access our empowered no, as we discussed in chapter 4, and the wave of compulsions will evaporate. At other times, the urge to be compulsive will grow stronger, but it will be amenable to negotiation. Then there will be times when our compulsion will be absolutely adamant. We can then choose to be compulsive, entering the wave with curiosity and gaining many valuable pieces of information all the way through.

During the wave. After that first puff of a cigarette or the bliss of chocolate melting in your mouth, the chant of "more, more, more" kicks in, and our urges get out of control. Rather than being lost in our compulsion, this is the time to recognize what we are doing. "Here I am," our awareness says, "in the middle of a wave of compulsion, caught in reaction and trying to deaden my feelings again. This always makes me feel worse in the long run." Recognizing that getting lost in our compulsion has never brought us the peace we long for gives us the courage to meet the feelings that are causing us to be compulsive in the first place. For it is guaranteed that if we are trying to distract ourselves through compulsion, the feelings that fuel it are very close to the surface. If we can be present for these feelings, even for a moment or two, they begin to transform back into the free-flowing energy they came from and no longer fuel our compulsions.

After the wave has passed through. After a wave of compulsion has passed through us is when we are most open to acknowledging that compulsions never bring us the peace that they promise. As the cravings have subsided enough for us to feel ourselves again, instead of paying attention to the price we pay for taking care of ourselves in this way, we usually get caught in self-judgment: "I did it again!" and despair: "I will never stop!"

When we're sidetracked in this way, we don't allow ourselves to experience the truth that compulsions take away much more than they give. We may know this intellectually, but to feel with great clarity what happens after a wave moves through allows us to face the truth that this behavior leaves only devastation in its wake. This is true whether we're left with the discomfort of a food hangover, the guilt of unskillful sexuality, the cloud of fear after a buying spree, or the imbalance in our body from drinking too much. Then when compulsions cast their spell again, promising that if we follow them they will give us all the comfort and peace we long for, we can remind ourselves of the price we will pay for believing them.

Some compulsions don't seem to come in clear and concise waves — you may feel that you overwork all the time or perceive yourself as a constant worrier. You can still have moments when you recognize that you are paying a heavy price for being compulsive in this way, and this is valuable information.

Transformation

Imagine what you would feel if you could transform your anxiety, anger, and despair into the aliveness of joy. Imagine what it would be like if you found a tool that could clear up your most challenging feelings just as the morning sun dispels the fog. That tool is curiosity. Cultivating the pure attention of curiosity is an amazing alchemical process, turning the base metals of all that we don't like about our lives into the gold of clarity and joy. It can transform the darkest of emotional states and even the cruelest of thoughts. This happens when we learn how to bring the light of compassionate attention first to the act of compulsion and then to the deep feelings that fuel it.

I call this process, which we'll explore in part 4, "treasure hunting," for when we can be present for what is happening with our compulsions, we discover the treasures that have always been hidden in their depths. For now let me share a story that will give you a glimpse into how the light of curiosity can transform not only our relationship to our compulsions but also the feelings that are fueling it.

I was working with a client who had seen the futility of trying to control her eating but hadn't yet learned how to bring the healing light of attention to whatever she was experiencing. Having had a falling-out with her father, she hadn't talked to him in quite a while. It was through a friend of the family that she discovered that he was sick. Her first thought was, "I don't want to deal with this. I have done all the healing that I want to do with him, and I will forget I even heard that he was ill."

As much as the mind believes that it can compartmentalize experiences, it can't. It is like telling a jury to disregard the supposedly inadmissible fact that the defendant has killed other people in the past. Two days after hearing about her father, my client noticed a very heavy feeling in her chest. Not yet having the skill of paying attention, she ignored it, hoping it would go away. That night she found herself lost in a huge wave of compulsion, and by the time she arrived at my office the next day, the gist of her words was, "When am I going to stop this bad behavior?" As she examined her experiences leading up to this binge, the information about her father came out.

In the safety of our relationship, the heaviness in her chest revealed itself again, along with a deep resistance to experiencing whatever feelings were behind it. Rather than allowing her to run away this time, I invited her to close her eyes and bring her attention to her body, describing what she found there. Immediately she took a deep breath and the whole experience lightened as she met the sensations of a tight chest and a band of tension in her throat. With the safety of pure attention, healing tears flowed as she experienced a lifetime of grief from having an unavailable father.

Not only did her attention free these boxed-up feelings, it also brought her important information straight from the heart of her experience. She could see the validity of her grief and understand that it was one of the core feelings that fueled her waves of compulsion. When she met the depth of sadness that resided in her chest, her relationship with her binge changed. Rather than judging it, staying caught in a cycle of self-hatred and despair, she understood why she had binged in the first place. This awareness left her spacious and merciful with herself and much more willing to be curious when she was compulsive. Now that she knows the power of curiosity, she will be able to be attentive to these feelings without needing to numb herself with a binge.

One of the deepest joys of cultivating curiosity is that after having brought deep awareness into the hidden parts of yourself, when they come to visit again you will be able to choose whether to identify with them or to let them go. For where there is awareness there is choice, and where there is choice there is freedom. Just imagine being in the middle of a busy day at work, one in which your most reactive state of mind is beginning to take over. And instead of getting caught in the maze of reaction, you recognize what you are experiencing and easily say, "I don't need to go there. I can let this go." That is the place that curiosity can bring us to.

Or imagine being in the middle of an argument, feeling anger toward the other person and in a flash recognizing that you are getting caught up in your outrage. Immediately, through the spaciousness of your awareness, you can let go of your anger and can instead be fully present with the other person. If that's not joy, I don't know what is. I have been in arguments like this in which my companion and I ended up laughing at how stuck we can get. Through curiosity not only can we transform our entrenched patterns back into joy, but we can also, when they come for temporary visits, immediately choose not to identify with these old states. In fact, we can let them go.

Awakening the Wellspring

Imagine what it would be like to know with absolute certainty that you are not alone. And imagine what it would be like to be in contact with a source of wisdom within you that guides you every step of the way. This is the healing that compulsions bring you — nothing less than a partnership with the wisdom at the heart of life.

Remember what it was like in the house of your being where, in the dark and fertile basement, you came across the circular room? As its walls dissolved, revealing a place of such lush beauty and flowing water, you probably felt pure joy. Well, that is not just a wonderful fantasy. That is what you discover on the journey back to yourself. There is a wellspring of wisdom within each of us that is the source of our deepest knowing. When we are in contact with its healing presence, we can accept ourselves as we are — both our strengths and our weaknesses. We can also trust ourselves and life, for inherent in our wellspring is an inner radar that can guide us skillfully through our lives. People call it a gut feeling, but it is much more than that. It is a grounding in ourselves and in life.

The seat of this wellspring is our belly. For thousands of years, some of the wisest teachers from the East have talked about this deep knowing within our bellies. Some call it *hara*. Some call it *tan tien*. Even Western scientists talk of the "abdominal brain." But most of us in the West are lost in our heads, lost in ideas about how our lives should be. Because our center of gravity is in our heads, we are not grounded in our bodies and thus are unable to listen to the wisdom there. Every time we bring our attention out of what was and what will be and instead become curious about what we are experiencing right now, we awaken our inner wellspring. Every time we *feel* our body rather than think about it, we energize this wellspring.

No matter how confusing our lives are or how lost we feel, our wellspring is waiting for us in the basement of our being. It may be blocked from view by all the boxes of hidden feelings we have stashed down there, but it is still there. Through our ability to be curious, along with the four questions we will be exploring in part 4, we can clear the boxes and connect with our wellspring again.

Practices for Awakening Our Curiosity

The beauty of curiosity is that it is so simple. You don't need to do anything except pay attention. Once you have made contact with what is happening inside you, you don't need to change what you discover there. You don't need to figure out where it came from or try to get rid of it. Your focused attention is enough. In fact, it is more than enough. It is nothing less than the alchemical transformer of life. This drives the corn maze of the mind crazy for a while because it is so used to doing *something* to stop the behavior! Healing doesn't come from changing anything. It comes from the relationship itself — from the ability to be present for exactly what is happening. And in this presence, right actions — healing actions — will reveal themselves. Can you remember a time when you were upset about something and somebody just listened to you? She hardly needed to say a word, and yet something lifted inside of you after being heard. That lifting comes from the power of focused attention.

Below I offer some practices to help you learn this invaluable skill of cultivating curiosity. As you explore these practices, notice what is being offered and work with what interests you. Some practices will call to you, and others won't. Trust your instincts. As you do, your unique way back into curiosity will reveal itself.

A Returning Practice

To gather the gifts of curiosity, we need to strengthen the muscle of our attention. This is what I call a Returning Practice, and it is very simple. It is about choosing a focus and then returning to it whenever your attention is captured by the thoughts in your head. Anything can be a focus — sounds, a pain in your knee, the taste of your food, or the rising and falling of your breath. Let us explore what this is like in the following exercise, using the sounds of life as our focus:

Exercise

After you read this paragraph, put down the book and close your eyes for a few minutes, listening as if you have just arrived on planet Earth. Every sound is brand new, coming straight from the heart of mystery. Be fascinated. This is the music of your life. Hear loud sounds and soft sounds. Hear the ones that are close and the ones that are far away. Whenever you notice that you are not listening to the sounds, without judgment return your attention to them. If your attention wanders a lot, count how many different sounds you hear. When you are ready, open your eyes.

As you do this exercise, you will notice that at times you will be purely present for the sounds of your life. Then your attention will slip back into the thoughts in your head. Notice this without judgment. Every time you bring your attention back to the sounds, you strengthen the muscle of your attention. The more you do this, the stronger it will become, increasing your ability to be curious about *what is*. It also becomes easier to see that there is a very big difference between being caught in ideas about life and actually experiencing it. People are often amazed when they first begin a Returning Practice to recognize not only how busy their mind is with nonessential things but also how an unattended mind has a tendency to wander all over the place, often getting itself into trouble!

The key to a Returning Practice is to know that your attention will drift off into your thoughts over and over. Big surprise! You have only been lost in thought for most of your life. The mind loves to think about life's dramas rather than experiencing what is happening right now. The healing of a Returning Practice isn't in staying on the focus. It comes from the willingness to return. And it is important to return gently. There is no need to judge how lost you get in your mind or to jerk yourself back.

Just as you make time to go to the gym to strengthen your muscles, it is helpful to set aside time every day for strengthening the muscle of your attention. For most of you, what will work best is just a few minutes every morning before your day and your mind begin to pick up speed. Find a quiet spot in your house where you won't be interrupted. Sit comfortably with both feet on the ground and with your spine as straight as possible. Then close your eyes and choose one focus. It could be listening to the sounds around you, paying attention to the rising and falling of your breath, or noticing the beating of your heart. Be willing to return to your focus over and over again whenever you find your attention drifting off. Start with five minutes, and as the muscle of your attention becomes stronger, try extending the time.

As you become more willing to cultivate pure attention I invite you to begin your daily Returning Practice by describing the space you are in — the colors you notice, the sounds, the shapes, the dance of shadow and light. The next step is to pay attention to your body. Notice the many sensations that are always present — warmth, coolness, tingles, pressure, pain, pleasure, aches, tickles. To be this present with your body is a little more intimate than paying attention to the space you are in. As your capacity to pay attention increases, eventually you will be able to go *inside* yourself and recognize exactly what you are experiencing in both your feelings and thoughts.

Know that you won't do this perfectly. Some days it will be easier to stay with your focus than others. As one of my teachers once said, "If you sit for an hour and only return to your focus once in that hour, it is time well spent." Of course that is an exaggeration, but it invites you not to judge how you are doing or even how you are progressing. Just be willing to return. Know that a few moments of returning your attention to exactly *what is* will transform your life in ways that your heart deeply longs for.

Returning throughout the Day

If you aren't inclined to sit with your eyes closed, choose one thing to do every day, and do it with curiosity. It could be your morning shower, when you focus on the sensations of the water cascading down your back, the tingle of your skin under the roughness of the washcloth, and the sweet smell of the soap. Ask yourself over and over, "In this moment, what am I experiencing?" (We will work more with this question in chapter 12.) Every time the mind goes off into the past or the future, bring it back into curiosity about the sensations of the shower.

We can make a Returning Practice out of almost anything in our lives. You could take a deep breath at every stoplight, experiencing it as fully as you can. Or you could choose your morning walk or run, coming back to the experience of your feet making contact with the earth. Every time I use the bathroom, I wash my hands with full attention. At moments it may seem like returning to the sensation of water on your back while taking a shower or the rising and falling of your breath won't help to transform anything in your life. Don't discount the power of even a few moments of *returning* during the day. Those moments are like drops of water that eventually become a trickle, then a stream, and finally a whole river of awakening that brings you the healing you so long for.

Whether you sit quietly every morning returning to a focus or you choose a focus to return to throughout the day (or both!), moments of pure attention teach you how to make contact with life, a contact for which you are deeply hungry. Focusing your attention and then returning when you drift away will teach you how to listen, to discover that all the clues to your healing are in the experience you are having right now. Focusing and returning also show you how to relax into the present without trying to fill it up with endless details. Finally, they reveal how to let go of the reactive mind that keeps you caught on the pendulum of control, moving you to the responsive mind that knows how to make kind and skillful choices.

Watching Your Story

We need to be gentle as we invite ourselves to be curious, for we have been caught in our struggling minds for a long time. But remember, in the beginning the power is in returning, not in staying on the focus. The more you return, the more fascinated you become by what *is* rather than by what was or what will be. You then become interested in discovering what keeps you apart from an alive and joyous engagement with life. What thoughts are so compelling that they feel more important than being present? It is possible to cultivate enough curiosity that you can see all the familiar struggles in your head rather than being lost in them. And when you can see them, you have a far greater chance of responding with skillful choices rather than reacting compulsively.

In the beginning, this can be a little bit like trying to see your face without the benefit of a mirror. You have been so close to your thoughts that it is hard to see what they are doing. To create space, you can add a wonderful technique to your Returning Practice. This technique will help you begin to develop the part of you that can see your thoughts rather than always being lost in them.

Exercise

Close your eyes and choose a focus. It could be the sounds of life appearing and disappearing all around you, or it could be the rising and falling of your breath. After grounding in your focus, when you notice that you are again lost in thought, take a moment before you return to your focus to notice whether your thoughts are about the past or the future. Squeeze your left hand and say "past" silently to yourself whenever you notice yourself thinking about the past, and then return to your focus. Squeeze your right hand and say "future" whenever you notice you are paying attention to the future, and then return to your focus. If it takes more than a split second to recognize past or future, or if you find yourself just spacing out, squeeze both hands and say "thinking, thinking" and then return to your focus.

This practice teaches you how to be curious about what your mind is doing. As your curiosity deepens, whenever you become distracted you can take this ability to watch your thoughts to even a deeper level. This happens by naming exactly what your thoughts are doing. What you are most likely to see going in your head are *planning, remembering, fearing, wanting, struggling, judging,* and just *spacing out.* The mind engages in myriad other activities, but these labels will give you a start. When you see what the mind is doing, note that action silently to yourself by saying it twice (like "planning, planning") and then return to your focus. Again, if it takes more than just a split second to see what is going on, simply say "thinking, thinking," and return to your breath.

The more you watch what your thoughts are doing, the more you come to realize that what passes through your head all day long is a story *about* life rather than a full and immediate experience *of* life. This story has grown throughout your life, with the experiences of your youth creating the core themes. The more you watch the story, the more your heart opens to how much wanting and fearing you have experienced in your life. And the more your heart opens, the more you realize this truth: you can see the story, *but you are not the story itself.* This is the freedom that our compulsions bring us.

Being Present for Yourself

As we stabilize our attention into moments when we can truly recognize life, right here, right now, we then feel that deep longing to truly meet ourselves — to be present for ourselves as we are rather than living in the endless story of how we should be. Let's explore what this feels like.

Exercise

When your attention is stabilized, broaden your focus by including your whole body. Ask yourself the question, "In this moment, what am I experiencing?" Your body is a constantly changing river of sensation, and it is different now than at any other moment in your life.

After you read through this exercise, take a few deep breaths and close your eyes. If your mind becomes easily distracted, stay with some deep breathing, allowing your body to melt with every out-breath. Without wanting to change anything, be curious about what you are experiencing and speak the truth of it silently to yourself. Are you warm or cold? Is your body comfortable or uncomfortable? Is there any pain in your body? Are there any pleasant sensations? Can you feel tingles, pressure, moistness? Stay with this for a few minutes, naming to yourself what you are experiencing. Then let your attention stabilize on the rhythm of your breath, riding the waves as they swell and recede. When you are done, open your eyes.

The technique is that simple. But do not be fooled by its simplicity. *In these few moments you were present for yourself.* You weren't trying to change yourself, and you weren't expecting yourself to be any different from what you are. This is one of the most powerful gifts you can give to yourself — your undivided attention. Tuning into exactly what is going on closes the gap between who we think we should be and who we really are, a priceless gift. This ability to check in and discover what is going on also keeps our bodies open and alive. And, most important, it keeps us from heading to the refrigerator, our credit cards, the bar, and so on.

Weather Reporting

We have spent our lives running away from our boxed-up feelings and habitual thought patterns, so we have to be patient as we learn how to turn toward ourselves again. As we shine the light of curiosity onto our immediate experience, it is helpful to speak the truth to ourselves about what we are experiencing. I call this Weather Reporting, for our experience is as variable and as uncontrollable as the weather. Just as a meteorologist doesn't try to create or change the weather, when we check in with ourselves we are reporting on what is happening, not trying to make it be different from what it is.

Weather Reporting allows you to relate to what is happening rather than becoming lost in it. And each time you speak the truth of what you are experiencing, you are no longer completely identified with it and have begun to disentangle yourself from its web. You can speak the truth of your experience either silently or out loud. When you are lost in a reactive state of mind it can be very powerful simply to acknowledge where you are. You can even do this when you are confused about what your experience is, for the truth in that moment is that you can't see what your experience is!

If you can understand that Weather Reporting isn't about changing anything, you will begin to get a glimpse of how powerful it is to speak the truth of your own experience, claiming what is going on without the need to judge, fear, or change it. I find I do this a lot while driving. If something is bothering me, I start by asking the question, "In this moment, what am I experiencing?" I then bring my attention back to my immediate experience, and, because I have been doing this for a number of years, it is fairly easy to see what is going on. Since I don't need to struggle with it, everything calms down quite quickly, and I am again in contact with my inner wellspring of wisdom.

It can also be helpful to bring what we are noticing inside us out into the light of day. We can do this either by writing down what we are experiencing or by speaking it to another person. One of the most powerful ways to write down our experiences is keeping an Awareness Diary. In this diary we make three columns on a piece of paper. We put on top of the first column *What is taking place right now?* On top of the second column we put *What is happening with my compulsion?* On the third column we write *What am I experiencing inside?* As an example let's use the challenge of trying to get all your holiday decorating done in just one day. As the day progresses and you can't find all your decorations, you've burnt two batches of cookies, and your kids don't want to cooperate, you find yourself heading down the slippery slope of your compulsion. Rather than staying unconscious, you pull out your Awareness Diary and write in the first column "holiday decorating." In the second you put down "starting to sneak food." In the third column you take a few moments, listen within, and then write "deep frustration, a building anger, and fleeting sadness."

You keep the diary on the table where you can make notes of what is happening both inside and outside you throughout the day, and you find this deeply comforting. Rather than falling into the unconsciousness of your compulsion, you are cultivating the consciousness of being present for your experience by writing it down.

I saw the full benefit of keeping an Awareness Diary when a woman in one of my groups began to keep track of her food intake. At first it was very difficult for her to record what she was eating, because every time she had done this before, it was to try to control her input of food. This time she was writing it down simply to become aware of what was going on. When she began noting what was happening internally and externally when she was eating, she could see some ancient patterns that were running her. A quick look back over the weeks and months clearly showed her the times when it was easiest for her to get triggered and what calmed her down again. The diary also moved her out of judging what she was doing into a much more compassionate relationship with herself.

We can also write our experiences in the way that Julia Cameron suggests in her book *The Artist's Way*.[3] With this kind of writing you allow the pen to move across the page continuously so that the censor in your head doesn't stop the flow. The more you do it the more you become connected to yourself. You discover parts of you that have never had a voice. Not only do they get heard, but you get to hear the wisdom that they have been trying to share with you for years. Julia suggests you do this every morning as a self-nourishing practice. You can also do it whenever and wherever you are in reaction to life, especially when you are compulsive. Grab the nearest piece of paper and start writing down what you are noticing. When you go back later and read what you have written, you will discover a treasure trove of information and insight about your internal experiences.

You can also weather report with another person, either a friend or a counselor. This person is your listening partner. She is not there to fix you, to change you, or to help you to understand anything. She is there to simply and profoundly listen. As you speak the truth of your experience, you are being heard and you are creating space in which to hear yourself. The benefit of choosing a counselor is that counselors are more likely to be trained in the art of listening. The benefit of choosing a friend is that friends are usually more available when challenges come up.

It is very important to choose wisely the person to whom you speak your truth. This person needs to understand the power of pure listening. Just as we don't listen to weather reports to change the weather, this person shouldn't try to make you be different. If you don't have someone in your life that knows how to do this, you may need to educate your listener. Before you speak, tell this person that all you want is deep listening and acknowledgment of what is being heard. Ask the person to refrain from giving advice, offering pity, or expressing judgment in any way.

This person also needs to be someone you can trust. You need to check this out with him before sharing. This trust includes that person's commitment never to speak to another about what you share unless you give your permission. It also includes his commitment not to judge you for what you will be revealing. These commitments create the safety you need to discover that you have practically every possible thought and emotion available to a human being. If you can speak the truth of what you are experiencing without fear of judgment or gossip, not only will you be heard, but you will also be returned to the place of true healing, which is the compassionate recognition of your own experience.

Whether you choose a friend, a counselor, or both (why not? You deserve it!), the key to speaking your truth and discovering the space to listen to yourself is in letting go of beginning a sentence with the words *I am*. When you say "I am sad," or "I am mad," or "I am hurting," you narrow your perception of yourself to just those experiences and lose perspective in the process. A better way to put it is "My body is," "My emotions are," or "My mind is." This slight linguistic shift creates space where you can *relate to* what is happening rather than *being lost in it.* This shift from *I am* to *it is* allows greater freedom. You are so much more than your experiences. The core of you is awareness itself — the ability to see *what is.*

I also invite you to weather report as you read this book. I am not offering you a cure. That is the old style of thinking in which your healing happens sometime in the future. This process is about inviting you into relationship with what is right now, for that is where true healing lies. This book will empower you, and it will confuse you. It will bring waves of joy and sometimes waves of fear. It may reveal distrust and self-judgment along with hope and mercy. In fact, it is designed to do so. Every experience you have in reading this book is a part of your healing, and it can be helpful to name to yourself over and over what is happening inside you as you read.

When we acknowledge our truth we retrain our attention so that when a seemingly unacceptable part of us makes itself known, we can turn toward it rather than away. This dramatically lessens its power over us — it is the doorway out of struggle. A moment here and a moment there spent listening to ourselves *as we are* rather than as we wish ourselves to be allows us to discover that we are fine just as we are, right now.

Learning to be curious so that we can be intimately and passionately present is an unfolding process, the work of a lifetime. Along the way we gather patience, compassion, trust, and the willingness to show up for the lives we have been given. The payoff is nothing less than rediscovering the rapture of being fully alive. So I invite you to cultivate moments of pure attention throughout your day. Be curious about what is happening inside you and outside you, knowing that in each moment of curiosity you are healing not only your own life but also the world.

Core Ideas

- The healing power of curiosity is that it invites us to stop striving for results and to start meeting things as they are.

- Curiosity is focused attention. It is neither for nor against whatever it focuses on. It is simply interested in what is happening right now. Its beauty lies in its simplicity, yet it is powerful beyond our ordinary comprehension.

- Through curiosity you can learn to bring the light of compassionate attention first to the act of compulsion and then to the deep feelings that fuel it.

- The more you watch what your thoughts are doing, the more you come to realize that what passes through your head all day long is a story *about* life rather than a full and immediate experience *of* life. Right beneath your busy, busy mind is a world of ease, aliveness, wisdom, and love.

- A Returning Practice will strengthen the muscle of your attention. The key is knowing that your attention will drift off and that healing comes from your gentle willingness to return to your focus.

- The healing power of Weather Reporting, using the question "In this moment, what am I experiencing?" lies in speaking the truth of what you are experiencing right now without any need to judge or change it.

Chapter 8

....

SKILL TWO:

LOVING OURSELVES FROM THE

Inside Out

efore I got up to speak at a four-day conference in the beautiful Cascade Mountains of Washington State, I looked across the aisle, and there, nestled in her mother's arms, was Emily. This image of a child totally safe in the world and completely loved touched me deeply. As the program on stage began, I kept turning my head and drinking in this nourishing image. Soon Emily noticed my gaze, and we began a love affair with our eyes that quickly developed into dancing, laughter, and hugs.

Matthew Fox was the keynote speaker, and the next day I felt compelled to attend his talk. This was a bit unusual for me because when I am teaching at a conference, I usually treasure my quiet time. Fox spoke from his heart, moving us into a passionate willingness to hold our vision for the world. He then had us dance this vision, and there was Emily beside me, so alive and so free. She reminded me of my own aliveness before I became withdrawn and frozen as a child.

After we had danced, Matthew had us get down on our knees with our foreheads on the floor and wail for all the unconsciousness of the world — our collective rage, bigotry, arrogance, self-judgment, and so on. About a minute into it, I had the urge to sit up, and there was Emily, with tears streaming down her face, weaving through all the kneeling people, desperately looking for her mother. As she headed toward me, I put my arms out, but at the last moment she veered off in search of mama. I felt a wave of grief that almost knocked me over. It only lasted for a few moments until the relief that came as I saw Emily's mom lift her right arm as if it were a wing and scoop Emily underneath her in an act of true mothering. Tears poured down my cheeks, tears of grief at not being able to comfort her and tears of joy at seeing her comforted.

I realized with stunning clarity that this was a metaphor for my own life. For most of it, I had wandered in disconnection, desperately looking for some place where I could rest in love. The grief was not only over all the times I felt so isolated and alone; it was also over all the times that I was unable to be present for myself. The relief I felt came from knowing how to lift my wing and enfold myself in my own heart no matter what was happening.

On that floor, with the voices of hundreds of people crashing all around me, my heart opened. I let in all the love that my struggling, judging, fearing mind had separated me from for so long. Rivers of love moved through my whole body as tears of joy cascaded down my face. Ah, the healing of the heart, the healing of acceptance, the healing of love. For those few moments I remembered the joy of loving myself from the inside out, letting in the love that is at the heart of existence.

For thousands of years people from all parts of the globe have spoken and written about what it is like when the truth of love unfolds from the deepest part of themselves, filling them with its radiance. They all say that it is like coming home. By *love*, I don't mean what most people mean when they use that word. Rather, I am pointing to the essence of our *being*, the source of the wellspring within us, the truth at the heart of existence.

In this chapter we will be exploring the third skill, Loving Ourselves from the Inside Out. We will learn how to allow the truth of love into our lives. It is not just some chosen few who can know this love; it is the birthright of every human being. To know the love that is the essence of life is why we are here. But like so many of us, for most of my life I didn't have a clue about the truth of love. Even when I began to get an inkling of what was there, right beyond my struggling mind, I was like a child who had lost the capacity to reach out and touch it.

What Separates Us from Love

Love is accepting and honoring. It is allowing and understanding. *It sees what is without any need to change it.* Rather than dividing things, it brings them together in harmony, whether they are our families, parts of the world, or parts of ourselves. Its power to heal is phenomenal. Why, when love is our birthright, do most of us live so apart from its healing presence? One of the main reasons is that we have been trained in its exact opposite. Instead of being taught how to be in a loving relationship with ourselves, we have been trained to struggle, dominate, judge, and compare. We believe that when we "get it together" we will know the love that we long for — both inside and out. This is the *I am not/I should be* style of relating to ourselves that causes such pain. Remember in grade school the red pencil marks that were all over your schoolwork, saying "excellent," "good," "fair," or "poor"? The power of that red pencil to determine how we perceived ourselves was so great!

In childhood we are taught to read and write, to ride a bicycle, and to do our chores, but *we are not taught how to be okay with ourselves as we are.* So we become ongoing projects to ourselves, focusing on what needs to be different rather than meeting ourselves as we are in the vast regions of our hearts. There is nothing wrong with wanting to better ourselves. But for most of us it becomes our primary mode of existence, causing us to miss the "enoughness" that we are right now. It also makes our lives so challenging. There are many difficulties we all have to face, and without knowing how to meet ourselves with understanding and mercy, we wound ourselves instead. Eventually the wounds weave a layer of scar tissue around our hearts.

If you doubt that, go back to a time where you made a big mistake. It may have been on the job or in your relationship. Choose a mistake for which you believe you were to blame. Then reconstruct how you related to yourself after that experience. If you are like most people, and if you are honest, you would have to say that you beat up on yourself unmercifully. This doesn't just happen with the big mistakes of our lives. Imagine being on an interview for a job that you really want. Can you feel the knot in your stomach? That is the endless knot of *trying* that comes from never learning how to value and accept yourself as you are.

Often this urge to better ourselves isn't very evident. It is there, nonetheless, as a subtle, quiet unease deep within, keeping us caught in a vicious circle of trying and failing. The more we expect ourselves to be better or different from what we are, the more we judge how we are doing. The more we judge, the thicker the scar tissue around our hearts becomes. The more disconnected we become from understanding and mercy, the more we expect ourselves to be different. It seems there is no escape from this no-win situation.

If self-judgment is allowed to run rampant through our minds and hearts it can solidify into shame. Self-judgment says, "I did it wrong." Shame says, "I am wrong." To live a shame-based life is agonizing, one of the most corrosive experiences a human being can have. When we live this way, essentially we are rejecting ourselves. To be filled with shame is to wake up every morning to a person you don't like, and that person is you! Imagine what it would be like to be locked in a room twenty-four hours a day, 365 days a year with someone you didn't respect and weren't keen to be with. That is what it is like to live filled with shame.

The key to healing the core of our shame is mercy. *Mercy* is such a wonderful word. It means "to refrain from harming; to relieve suffering." When we have mercy we understand that the most unacceptable parts of us are the most wounded. We also know that every part of us deserves to be met in a compassionate and merciful way. One of the core roadblocks to discovering mercy is the belief that if we were merciful with ourselves, we would never be enough. So we flail at ourselves hoping this will make us acceptable enough to get the love that we long for. Round and round we go, often hurting ourselves when we are hurt, rejecting ourselves when we need mercy, and abandoning ourselves when we most need to be met.

This dynamic was dramatically illustrated in an episode of the television program *20/20 Downtown* in which a heroin addict and prostitute named Duran was interviewed. In a gravelly voice deepened and scarred by years of living on the streets, she eloquently spoke about her self-rejection. Her story gives us a glimpse into the self-rejection we all carry. When asked if she would ever give up drugs, she said, "I will never give up drugs. Giving up dope is confessing pain, and I am not going there because I have had too much goddamn pain in my life. I will never give up drugs as long as it means that I have to experience who I am in private. I am a hundred miles an hour on top of three or four hundred dollars of heroin a day, and that buffers me down just enough to the level I can deal with who I am."[1]

Even though we may not be prostitutes or heroin addicts, on some level we all have difficulty accepting ourselves as we are, especially the parts of us that are in pain. Cut off from our own mercy, each of us carries, in the deep regions of our being, a desperate longing for the warmth of a tender heart. Into this longing for understanding, exacerbated by self-judgment, come compulsions to numb and comfort our hurting hearts. We either use our compulsions to lessen the tension building inside us, or we use them to grab hold of some sense of ease that seems so far away. All these things keep us very far from a kind and loving relationship with ourselves.

The Schoolroom of the Heart

It is possible to open our hearts again, learning how to meet ourselves in understanding and mercy. It is possible to love ourselves from the inside out so we can know again the love that is at the heart of everything. It is not only possible; it is what healing is all about. This is one of the core treasures that our compulsions bring us. They won't let us go until we see that acceptance heals. They will show us over and over again that all our fixing, judging, and rearranging has never brought us the peace that we long for.

We will return to an abiding and ease-filled connection with ourselves and with life only through accepting ourselves as we are. As Sri Nisargadatta Maharaj, a respected spiritual teacher from India once said, "The mind creates the abyss; the heart crosses it."[2] Acceptance is so powerful that it can heal bodies, relationships, even nations. Do you want to heal yourself? For just this moment accept yourself as you are. Do you want to help heal your family? For just this moment accept yourself as you are. Do you want to help heal the world? For just this moment accept yourself as you are.

To cultivate moments when we allow ourselves to be just as we are is not lazy or weak. In fact, it is the most courageous thing we can do. It allows us to be more productive, because we are living from our truth. To fall in love with ourselves is not selfish — it is one of the most selfless gifts a human being can give to the world. *If you can accept yourself as you are, you can accept others as they are.* You then become a healing presence in the world.

Learning how to love ourselves and then live from our inner wellspring is what life is all about. To help you grasp this truth, I invite you to take a trip up to the moon with me:

You will find a cozy armchair up there where you can sit down and reflect on life from a broader perspective. I ask you to suspend all judgment until the end of this section and feel what I am saying here. As you settle in, you see the Earth before you in all its beauty. See the blues of the rivers and oceans, the whites of the snowy peaks and fluffy clouds, the gold of the rolling hills, and the green blankets that pour across the continent. All this is framed against the black, velvety backdrop of space. Take a moment and be stunned. And if your heart hasn't yet gotten how miraculous your home is, look over at Mars, beautiful in its own right, but basically just red rock. Now look back at the Earth and be amazed by the creativity that has been able to flourish on this planet.

Our planet wasn't always this way. At its inception, it was nothing more than a roiling, boiling cauldron of gas and dust. Yet a river of creativity has flowed through time and has learned how to weave itself into waterfalls and iridescent wildflowers, dolphins and jaguars, wildly colored parrots dancing through orchid-covered trees, and a two-legged creature called a human being that populates almost every nook and cranny of the globe.

Why has life brought forth such creativity on this planet? None of us can ever really know the purpose of life — it is too big for our minds to comprehend. But we can make a guess; and I believe that when a guess comes close to the truth, it invigorates and inspires us. Of all the ideas I have tried on over the years, none has resonated so deeply as the idea of Earth as a schoolroom of the heart. It is a place to learn about love, to recognize love, and to live from love. In other words, we are all love waking up to the truth of love.

The best way to comprehend what we are exploring here is to recognize that every step of the way — from the gas and dust of the universe's beginning to the stupendous diversity of the oceans and the rivers to the air we breathe to the land that we walk on, even to you and me — was about life coming together into greater communities. From atoms to molecules, from molecules to cells, and from single cells to multicelled beings, this process has occurred. Every step of the way the components of life were being drawn together into greater wholes.

The best word I have ever heard used to describe this drawing together is *allurement*. The definition of *allurement* is "the power to attract." Another word for it is *love*. Love is the activity at the heart of life that draws molecules together to make rocks, cells together to make animals, and all forms of life together to procreate so this great river of creativity can continue to flow. Rumi wrote about this force field of love:

I have discovered Love!
How marvelous, how good, how beautiful it is!
I offer my salutation to the spirit of passion
that aroused and excited this whole universe
and all it contains.[3]

The love that Rumi speaks about is the allurement at the heart of life that holds it all together. This passion is bringing us all to the next great coming together. This isn't a physical coming together; it is a coming together in consciousness. It is a coming together of the community of life in the minds and hearts of human beings. It is the awareness of the oneness of all life and the living of this truth.

You and I have arisen out of the creativity of this planet. Each of us *is* the Earth. We may not have roots like a tree or fins like a fish, but we have been woven out of her mighty mountains, her rushing rivers, and her dancing wind. We have the oceans of the Earth coursing through our veins. Our bones are made out of particles of mighty mountains that have dissolved into us. We are each an animated piece of the Earth that has learned how to walk, talk, write, and sing. One of the core gifts we have been given is the ability to explore it all. The dolphins can explore only the seas; worms only the ground; gorillas only the forests. But we can travel from the highest of mountains to the deepest of seas and be awed by what we discover. From all our exploring, we can begin to see that we have very special gifts to give back to life:

- We can be moved in wonder by the vast creativity that was necessary in forging this planet and everything on it, including us. We can comprehend that it is possible for us to see, dance, laugh, think, and love because of all that has gone before us.

- We can recognize the beauty of absolutely everything. Nothing is ordinary! Even a straggly plant is an amazing creation.

- We can see that everything is necessary, weaving together the great tapestry that is the universe.

- We can celebrate that each particle of this planet is a unique expression of the creativity of life, never having been seen before and never to be seen again.

- We can also begin to see that we are all in this existence together, living on a tiny, fragile jewel that is floating through vast oceans of space.

You and I are nothing less than a part of life that can recognize and celebrate its stupendous creativity and its dazzling beauty. Let it in. Allow this vision of life to inspire your mind and open your heart. Love is calling to you, asking you to wake up to the wonder of life, to the miracle of you. You are enough. In fact, you are more than enough. You are a unique and necessary expression of life. And life is asking you to see the totality of yourself — all your strengths and your weaknesses, your joys and miseries — through the eyes of your heart. *For it is within your heart that you can weave all the parts of yourself back into the wholeness that is you.*

If you truly understand that you are a part of the Earth, then it becomes evident that as you heal, so too does the Earth. In the multitude of our human hearts, all life will be woven back into the whole that it is so that love can flourish on this planet. As Teilhard de Chardin, the beloved Jesuit priest once said, "Someday, after we have mastered the winds, the waves, the tides and gravity... we shall harness the energies of love. Then, for the second time in the history of the world, mankind will have discovered fire."[4]

Let us now explore how our compulsions can become our guides into loving ourselves, loving life, and allowing ourselves to be loved in return.

How Our Compulsions Teach Us to Love

This awakening to the essence of love that permeates life is taking place in the minds and hearts of individuals all over the world — including you. You are a part of it, and everything in your life is tailor-made to open you again so that you can do the most courageous, the most challenging, but also the most healing thing a human being can do — fall in love with yourself. The particular body you have been given, the type of personality you have, the family you were raised in, your work, and your community are all a part of your schoolroom of the heart. And your compulsion is your graduate course.

There is practically no better place to learn about self-acceptance than with our compulsions. They teach us how deeply we are disconnected from ourselves. Think about what happens right before a wave of compulsion hits. We usually feel a great deal of tension because of all the pressure we put on ourselves for not being okay as we are. Compulsions also bring to light how much we believe that self-judgment will whip us into shape. Think about what happens after a wave has moved through. Usually your heart is closed tighter than a drum and you are berating and belittling yourself for "screwing up again." Our compulsions trip us up over and over again, revealing the places where our hearts are closed to ourselves.

Compulsions also reveal to us the power of mercy and how deep our hunger for it is. They will bash us against the wall of control, judgment, and despair until we discover the tiny flicker of light from a merciful heart. We go to that light like a traveler lost in the night. The closer we get, the brighter it becomes until we crawl into its warm embrace and discover that it had always been waiting for us just beyond the prison of our closed hearts.

My compulsion was the only thing painful enough to shatter the illusion that I could *purchase* the love I longed for by making myself into an *acceptable* person. Caught in the endless maze of fixing, changing, managing, and controlling, I would numb myself when again I became lost in failure and self-rejection, hoping to get away from the pain of my closed heart. Yielding to my compulsion was also an attempt to alter my experience in the hopes that I could know a little of the joy that naturally exists when my heart is open. But usually this running away from what I was afraid of and this running toward the oblivion of compulsion brought only short relief before the self-cruelty began again.

It took me a long time to realize that this numbing out would never work and that it wasn't food that I was hungry for, but the tender understanding of my own awakened heart. Even if a friend or loved one met me with understanding and mercy, it was never enough. *It was my own heart that I was hungry for.* I finally had to face the fact that the person I really wanted to hear "I love you" from was me. My compulsions narrowed down my options until the only thing that was left was to meet myself *as I was.* Dropping out of my mind and back into my heart, I finally discovered the healing I longed for.

This view of compulsions may be a stretch for you, but just think about it for a moment. Has it ever really worked for you to treat your compulsion as the enemy and as proof that you are defective? Soften your stance for a moment and contemplate the idea that all the desperate wanting behind your compulsive activities is really a longing for tender self-acceptance. You've just never known how to meet yourself in that way. Allow in the deep knowing that heart energy circumvents the endless game of trying to solve our problems, and instead it dissolves those problems.

A number of years ago I had a revealing experience at a doctor's office. I was going through a time when my body was unbalanced and I was very uncomfortable. I was with an HMO at that time, so the doctor I went to for help was not one I would have chosen. While she was very learned, empathy was not one of her strong suits. As the appointment progressed, her coldness, along with the reality that there really was no cure for my beleaguered body, threw me back into that desperation of my childhood, and there to meet it was the old sadistic urge to reject myself.

"You are such a wimp," the bully inside of me said. "It doesn't matter that you can't raise your arms to comb your hair. It doesn't matter that you are running unexplained fevers. You always make a big thing out of nothing. Here you are doing it again and being such a bother." It was relentless, cunning, and almost engulfing. In the face of this self-cruelty, I wanted to run out of the office, straight to a grocery store, and inhale the first thing I came across. But because my compulsion had shown me that judging myself for being vulnerable and then falling into overeating only made it worse, I turned to acceptance, understanding, and mercy instead.

"These are old voices from the past," my awareness said. "I need to get out of here and meet them with my heart." I went to my car and took long, deep breaths. Even though I had been slowly removing the scar tissue from around my heart, it was still a place where the old bullying and belittling voices could get a temporary foothold and where compulsion could become interesting again. I closed my eyes and felt the knot of self-hate in the pit of my stomach. I said, "I recognize you. You are a visitor from my past. I give you my attention without believing what you have to say."

While I was exploring this sadistic urge to reject myself when I was the most vulnerable, my heart opened. Underneath these voices, I could feel the very scared part of me that was afraid it would never, ever feel better. This thought was irrational in relation to what was happening at that moment, but it wasn't irrational in relation to how it was created in my childhood, only to live on year after year.

Never in my life had I met this depth of vulnerability with an equal depth of understanding and compassion. I was no longer rejecting myself when I was scared, and I was no longer rejecting myself when I was rejecting myself! My closed heart was pointing the way toward opening, and thus the urge to compulsively stuff my face faded away, leaving me fully accepting of my thoughts, my feelings, and my body. Such sweet relief! No words describe the joy that floods your being when you meet a formerly hated and feared part of yourself with your heart. It leaves you spacious, alive, and so very glad to be given the gift of reconnecting with yourself. There is also no reason to run off to your compulsion, for there is nothing to run from and no comfort to run to. You are already giving yourself the comfort that you need — a merciful heart.

A few days after this experience, I went to the conference where I met Emily. She revealed to me the aliveness and joy that are always present behind the locked doors of my heart. Her presence also reminded me that my tears and my pain could now dance and sing in the safety of my own mercy.

An Invitation

Before we begin cultivating a merciful heart, we need to recognize that most people have at least some difficulty meeting themselves in mercy. For many it is almost impossible.

Exercise

To discover how capable you are of seeing yourself through the "eyes of your heart," I invite you, after reading these two paragraphs, to go to a mirror and not only look at yourself but really see yourself. Look beyond all those ancient beliefs that you are too much of this and not enough of that, and for these few moments recognize yourself. Don't get caught up in society's narrow idea of beauty. See yourself as you were created by life. Drink it in.

You are a totally unique expression of the mystery of life. You have been brought forth out of life's longing to express itself as you. If the old stories about "what could or should be better" try to take over, look beyond them and truly see yourself. And there you are, in all your glory, a magnificent, multifaceted, absolutely necessary expression of a great river of creativity. Now look into your eyes. There is you looking back at you. See yourself. Stay with this for at least a few moments, receiving yourself in all your depth.

Were you able to go to the mirror? Were you able to see yourself with respect and mercy? If not, know that you are in good company. Most people either would not look in the mirror in the first place or, if they did, all they would see is their defects. Many people who can make contact with themselves in the mirror still have difficulty acknowledging their own magnificence.

Know that whatever you could or couldn't do, it's okay. You are on the pathway back to reconnecting with yourself, with life, and with the love that you are. Everything grows and blooms in its own time and its own way, including you. One day you will recognize who you really are and rejoice in loving yourself from the inside out. So let us now explore some ways to open our hearts.

Practices for Opening Our Hearts

You can't force your heart open, but you can begin to cultivate an open heart. There are a million ways to do this, each one as unique as the person who created it. Below I offer a few techniques to get the ball rolling. Play with these skills only if they call to you. For, again, we come across a great paradox of life: we need to do everything that we can to open our hearts, *and* we need to understand that they are being opened by forces far greater than us. It is good to cultivate an open heart *and* to know that in the perfect time and the perfect way, even if it takes longer than you think it should, your life is bringing you back into a deep and loving relationship with yourself.

Watching Self-Judgment

The first step in returning to a spacious heart is *to notice how closed your heart is.* All of us experience a closed heart to some degree. We continuously conduct an inner conversation in which we're checking out how we are doing. For some, these voices are subtle. For others, they have solidified into shame and have become voracious demons. Most of us have some of each. But we all live, to a greater or lesser degree, with the idea that we need to be different from what we are to be okay. The truth is that trying to be *good* never brings us the results we desire, because being *good* is based on the supposition that we are *bad!* If we try to get rid of or run away from these voices in our heads, we stay stuck to them like glue. If we wake up to them instead, learning how to hear the voices in action rather than believing what they are saying, we are more likely to become free of their spell.

The first time I was able to observe the shaming voices in action inside me rather than believing what they were saying was a red-letter day. I had thought everything those voices said was the Truth. I bowed before these caustic and critical voices when they said, "I screwed up again. I will never get it right. Everybody else does it better than me. I am too fat, too stupid, too clumsy, too ugly, too needy, too selfish. I am too much of this and not enough of that." Of course I also got caught in the exact opposite views expressed by these voices: "I am better than you. I am smarter, more beautiful, skinnier (only when I was dieting!). And I don't need anybody, because I am above all that!" Ah, the pain that comes from believing those voices. And naturally compulsion served as a handy buffer between me and the pain of self-rejection. But only temporarily, for being compulsive always made it worse.

It took me a while to learn how to relate to these voices because they were so seductive. Most of the time, I experienced them as a foggy, relentless feeling of just not being okay. But at times they flared up into cruel monsters that wounded me to my core. It felt like they had written a doctoral dissertation on how to judge me. Not only that, they had also gotten a law degree so they could argue their case! As I discovered how to be free from these voices, I learned something I want to share with you: *They don't know what they are talking about! They are the result of ancient patterns in your head, and they don't have a clue about who you really are.* They are like an eight-year-old saying she knows how to run a corporation!

We can silence these voices of self-judgment and shame through a powerful but simple exercise called Watching Self-Judgment:

Exercise

For this exercise, carry around a little notebook, and whenever you catch yourself judging yourself, write down what the voice said. This is a very clarifying experience. When you see the words written on paper, it becomes easier to realize how cruel and ridiculous they are. This realization gives you the curiosity and the space you need not to fall under their spell. It is very important to realize as you do this that everybody else hears the same voices! Although it may not look like it on the surface, I guarantee that we all have a capacity to judge and shame ourselves to our core.

When I did this exercise, I took it one step further. I wrote the words spoken by the voices on a big piece of paper taped to a wall in my bedroom. As I looked at this paper, not only was I able to see the words more clearly, but I could also see the themes these voices were using. It took time, but eventually, when a voice screamed, "You never do anything right!" I was able to say to the voice, "Oh, you must be having a bad day!"

At first it can be scary to observe these voices. It's as if you're being asked to get into a cage with a man-eating tiger. When the voices are near, you can use a powerful statement to keep you from falling under their spell. Just say, "If it is unkind, it's of the mind." This statement reminds us that all the stories in our heads that put us down, no matter how seductive they are, are just old tapes. They are the result of learned patterns of relating to ourselves through expectation and judgment rather than from the vast healing of our hearts — and they don't know a thing about who we really are!

Listening Deeply

In exploring our self-judgment and shame, we will come across parts of ourselves that are difficult to accept. Not knowing that everybody else has his or her own unacceptable parts, our only option seems to be to reject ourselves. As long as we hide these objectionable parts from ourselves and the world, they will still have the power to make us believe that what they're telling us is true. They will also continue to fuel our compulsions from underneath our everyday awareness.

To open our hearts to these seemingly unacceptable parts, we can live in the question, "How can I bring compassion to this experience?" (a question we'll explore further in part 4). It can also be very helpful to find a person or a group with whom we can speak our truth. We find great healing when someone listens to our most unacceptable parts from a place of understanding and mercy. At first we may resist this, for we are absolutely certain that if somebody knew about these parts of us we would be thoroughly rejected. But the power of sharing our truth can be very healing.

Recently I was working with a woman who was on a trip with a friend from work. My client had been having panic attacks for a number of years. Because she was very ashamed of them, she had gone to great lengths to hide them from everybody, including her co-workers. Slowly and surely she was healing herself to her core. But since she was traveling, which is often stressful, some of the old feelings had resurfaced. She woke up the first morning with panic racing through every part of her. She was certain that to reveal what she was experiencing to her friend would be a disaster. But the more she tried to hide her panic, the worse it got. Finally the pain was so great that she shared her experience, expecting judgment in return. Instead, she received not only understanding but also a closer connection with her friend. Through her willingness to be real, she took another step into a compassionate connection with herself.

Being heard can break the cycle of hating and hiding, but we need to carefully choose our listening partner. As we explored in the last chapter, your partner needs to be a person or a group who won't judge you for your perceived imperfections and who won't broadcast what you say to the world. It also needs to be understood that you are not asking for opinions or advice: you just need to be heard. If you have never done this, you may not know the power of receiving complete, nonjudgmental attention. I assure you, it is far more powerful than anything you have done when you were busy fixing, changing, and rearranging yourself.

It is also helpful to make this practice into a two-way street. First one person listens in complete attention and trustful acceptance to whatever the other is experiencing, and then the other person listens. To listen while others share their vulnerability not only helps us understand that we are all in this together, but it also teaches us how to listen without judgment.

Since many of us have been caught in a glut of self-rejection, we might not have a friend or a group such as this. So we may need to contact a professional, such as a counselor or a minister. This is what I did at the beginning of my healing. There was no way I could speak my deepest hates and fears to friends or loved ones. I so completely hated my so-called defects that I absolutely knew and expected that I would be rejected if I shared them. If anyone so much as sneezed as I was expressing my deepest pains, I knew that the sneeze was an indication of his or her loathing of me!

Not only do people who have been listened to become healed, but they also become healers in the world. Being listened to shows them how to listen to themselves. And having learned how to listen to themselves, they can then be present with the grocery store clerk, the agitated bus rider, the rebellious teenager, the grieving loved one, and the scared child without turning it all into an emergency. A single moment of being present with another is a transformational moment for all of life.

Accepting Yourself as You Are

The first two practices we have just explored allow us to see and acknowledge how closed our hearts are so we can develop a relationship with ourselves based on understanding and mercy. For many people, the idea of loving themselves is too big a leap. It can feel so scary and alien that it shuts them down. So we need to take baby steps by first learning — for a moment here and a moment there — how to accept ourselves exactly as we are. Just as we needed to do addition and subtraction before we could do multiplication and division, we need to start with self-acceptance to learn how to love ourselves from the inside out.

Accepting ourselves comes from the understanding that all life is a dance of opposites. Nature needs the cold fury of winter in order to become the riotous blooming of summer. It needs raging lightning storms to ignite the fires that clear the forest for new growth. It needs volcanoes erupting from deep within the oceans to make new islands in paradise.

Just as life has interwoven the opposites of dark and light to birth itself into more creative expressions, it has done the same with us. We each have positive and negative attributes. Even though you are not a Hitler, you probably have been very cruel toward yourself in attempting to remake yourself into a perfect human being, in much the same way that Hitler tried to create what he perceived as a perfect race. Elisabeth Kübler-Ross, Swiss psychiatrist and author, as a take-off on the transactional analysis book *I'm OK, You're OK*, once jokingly said that she was going to write a book titled *I'm Not OK and You're Not OK and That's OK!* If we could even get a glimmer of how powerful it is to accept ourselves as we are, allowing our hearts to open, we would satisfy one of the deepest longings that we all feel — the longing to love ourselves.

We all have things we do well and things we don't. In fact, if you listed all the things that a human being is capable of, the odds are that you could probably only do a small percentage of them. Can you win the Tour de France five times? I thought not. How about wiggling your ears without moving any other muscles? The odds aren't with you. So there are far more things you can't do than you can! When we look at ourselves in this way, we see that we are nutty as fruitcakes and completely inept at most things. The only conclusion we can come to is that our perfection lies in our imperfection! One of the truest truths I have come across as the clouds in my mind have dissolved in the light of my heart is that, with all of the mistakes I have made, I never really made a mistake. Each one was a necessary part of the unfolding of my journey.

A wonderful image that illustrates this idea is an exquisitely woven tapestry. If you look at the underside, all you see are loose threads and lots of knots. The closed heart only lets us look at the bottom and misses the perfection of the weaving that shows on the other side. The open heart lets us look at both the top and the bottom and not only see the exquisite art work but also recognize the necessity of the jumble of threads and knots.

Do you feel relief at the thought that your imperfections are a part of your perfection? If we can accept that, then we can stop struggling so much. We can see that the most powerful way to learn about loving ourselves is to acknowledge what we don't do well. In fact, we have been given our weaknesses and vulnerabilities specifically as a training ground for the heart. We fall in love with ourselves as we learn how to embrace ourselves *as we are* rather than always trying to be what we think we should be. If we can grasp that for even a moment, our hearts can open just a little more, and we can take another step into loving ourselves from the inside out.

The wonderful thing is that we don't have to "get it together" to cultivate this type of relationship. In fact, it doesn't matter what is happening in our lives. We can do this when our hearts are completely closed, for we can open our hearts to how closed they are! If we are afraid to accept ourselves, we can accept our fear. If we are sure we are unworthy of this kind of love, we can accept our feeling of unworthiness. The key is accepting ourselves for whatever we are feeling and experiencing at this moment. *Whatever is happening is all right.* This is so effortless! It is occurring in the vast dance of dark and light that comprises life.

Because we have been trained to believe that fixing, changing, and rearranging ourselves will bring us the peace that we long for, hardly any of us knows how to tap into the powerful healing of acceptance. We haven't yet discovered that true acceptance is magic. Jon Kabat-Zinn, psychiatrist and author of *Full Catastrophe Living: Using the Wisdom of Your Body and Mind to Face Stress, Pain, and Illness*[5] began a pain clinic at Massachusetts General Hospital in the 1980s based on teaching patients how to be curious and accepting of whatever was happening in their bodies. The doctors sent him challenging cases figuring he would fail. Instead, he had phenomenal results that changed many people's lives, including the doctors'. Basically, he taught his patients not to fight pain. As they learned how to do this, many of them discovered that *most of their suffering was the result of resistance to their pain.* The power of softening around pain and accepting its presence brought so much relief that when they researched how many people were still using the techniques fifteen years later, most of them were.

The challenges in our lives can reveal to us the power of acceptance. I learned it through having a very sensitive body with a digestive tract that easily gets out of balance. There was a time when nothing I did seemed to make it any better. The doctors didn't have a clue about what to do, and neither did I. Besides being very uncomfortable, it brought up a lot of fear. One of the worst feelings was an almost constant queasiness that would flare up into nausea. If you saw me when I was reacting to this discomfort, you would have seen tight shoulders, a deep furrow in my brow, and a scowl on my face. For a long time, the only thing I knew how to do was react, lost in hate and fear of this unpleasant and scary experience. Needless to say, this always made it worse.

It took me a while, but out of desperation I learned how to go toward the experience — to open up around the nausea and actually be present with it. All I was doing was acknowledging the truth of my experience and then moving toward acceptance of it. When I wasn't fighting what was going on, the queasiness lessened, and sometimes it even left. The most important thing was that my whole relationship to the nausea changed, making it much easier to live with when it returned. In those moments when I could accept exactly what was happening rather than fighting it, I could act from a much wiser place.

As my body taught me that resisting what I was experiencing usually made it worse, it made sense to me that my feelings would also respond to acceptance. Over time, I learned that the very thing I was resisting, whether it was a physical feeling or an emotion, was the very thing I needed to accept. As I met all the various parts of myself in understanding and mercy, I began to accept the totality of who *I am!* — both the light and the dark. Let's practice this acceptance now:

Exercise

To taste the healing power of acceptance now, pause for a moment and think about something that you wish were not a part of your life. Start with something small, like a slight headache or irritation at your dog. Accept that it is a part of your life right now. Accept that life is not bad, and that you are not defective for having this experience. Take a few deep breaths and say to yourself, "For this moment, I let this be here." The flavor of this statement is acceptance. It says, "I accept that this is part of my journey right now. It's okay. I'm okay." You can amplify the statement by placing your hand over your heart.

Feel how acceptance softens your stance and makes everything more workable. This kind of acceptance isn't about being at the mercy of the challenges in our lives — it is about letting go of resisting them so that we can see the challenges through the clear eyes of our hearts. We then become able to act from wisdom rather than reaction.

I was working with a client once who had a very difficult boss. She often got lost in her fury at him. She also got lost in how furious she was for being furious! When she could accept that she felt rage over this person, she stopped fighting it, and her whole body softened. When she went back to work and the rage showed up, she wasn't surprised. She could even begin to have a little humor about it. Her willingness to accept her rage changed her entire work environment.

We have been deeply taught to resist our emotions, our pains, our lives, and ourselves. We react to our resistance, and then we react to our reactions. That is the world of struggle that we live in most all of the time. Yet one moment of acceptance is much more powerful than millions of moments of resistance. Take the question "For this moment, can I let this be here?" into your life. This is another one of the core questions we will be exploring in the Treasure Hunting part of the book. Another way you can say this is, "I accept that this is part of my life right now. It's okay. I'm okay." Use one of these statements whenever you find yourself resisting something. You will find that moments of acceptance can open your heart again, allowing you to live from the clarity, wisdom, and love that come from your truest self.

Making a Gratitude List

Another wonderful thing to do to open your heart is to make a list every day of three qualities you appreciate about yourself. Appreciation is the sunlight of human life, and a little bit goes a long way. Doing this is so powerful because we are trained to look at what is wrong with us, and it retrains us to look for what is right. When we start doing this, we see how often we have overlooked our own magnificence.

When I first started making a gratitude list on the advice of my counselor, I couldn't think of even one thing to write down. When I told him that I couldn't find a single good quality about myself, he asked if I had taken a shower before I came to see him.

I said, "Yes."

"Did you pick up the bath mat when you were done?" he asked.

I said, "Yes."

So the first item on my list was that I pick up bath mats. Now, that may seem like a very small thing, but it became a doorway into looking for what was right about myself rather than always focusing on what was wrong.

Making a gratitude list is about taking another step into your magnificence. Thomas Merton once said, "I have the immense joy of being human.... The sorrows and stupidities of the human condition can no longer overwhelm me, now that I realize what we all are. If only everybody could realize this! But it cannot be explained. There is no way of telling people that they are all walking around shining like the sun."[6] Even though there is "no way of telling people," I am telling you: you are beautiful beyond your wildest imagination. For this moment, let that in.

Let your heart open, and then write your list from that place of openness. You can even put Merton's quote on the top of each page of your notebook to remind you why you are making this list. Slowly, like a thousand veils lifting one after another, you will discover that you are *walking around shining like the sun!*

Really Seeing Yourself

As we explored earlier in the chapter, we can use our reflection both to open our hearts and to see how closed they are. As we move through our days, we encounter an abundance of mirrors and reflective surfaces where we can see ourselves. If we can move beyond the act of *looking* at ourselves to the act of *seeing* ourselves, we can take these moments to pause, connect, and open our hearts.

When I was first invited to see myself in mirrors, I was usually repulsed by what I saw. I went to amazing lengths to ignore the mirror while I brushed my teeth and even when I put on mascara. But I kept at it, and there were brief moments when I could see myself and keep my heart open. The first time a true dose of love wiggled its way into my perception was when I turned off the light by my bed late one night and saw my reflection in the window. Much to my amazement, my heart melted in tenderness, just as a lover's heart would. Oh, the joy of that moment. My heart was open to me! I now consciously cultivate that kind of connection with my reflection to keep the juices of respect and love flowing. Whenever I wash my hands, I always look into the mirror and say, "Hi." I sometimes even wink! I invite you to be willing to see yourself whenever you look into a mirror. This is not just a glance; this is looking at yourself in the curious and open way you would use when looking at the face of a lover or a child. And if seeing yourself brings up self-rejection, take your attention there and give that old voice a dose of tenderness and mercy.

When Your Heart Is Closed Tight

The techniques we have explored so far work when the door of our heart is open enough to let in the light of mercy. What do we do when our hearts are closed tight and we are absolutely sure that the mean and nasty voices are correct? We can use three techniques to open the doors again.

The Lost Child Meditation

This is a good exercise for discovering exactly what you need right now and then awakening your heart by giving whatever that is to an imaginary child inside you.

Exercise

Breathing deeply to calm your mind and body, close your eyes and imagine walking down a residential street. From a distance you hear the faint sounds of a child crying. As you come around the corner, you see the child sitting on the curb, crying her heart out. Imagine that whatever you are experiencing, she is experiencing the same thing.

If you are feeling all alone, imagine that her daddy has just moved out because of a divorce and she is heartbroken. If you feel very confused, not knowing your way out of a particular situation, imagine that she is lost and doesn't know her way home. If you find yourself hating yourself, imagine that all the neighborhood kids have just told this child that she is a dork and they don't want to play with her.

Allow your heart to open to her pain. Now imagine how you would comfort her. Then give that to her, whether it is a hug, a kind word, or a hand to hold. Experience the feeling of your heart touching hers in understanding and compassion. Whatever you imagined and whatever you felt is exactly what you want from you. Turn the light of this mercy toward yourself. Place your hand over your heart and give to yourself whatever you gave to this child. Say the words, imagine the touch, and feel this experience as deeply as you can. You are worthy of acceptance and love.

The Ball of Love Meditation

This powerful exercise can open the door to receiving love, reminding us that no matter what is happening in our lives, we are loved by life.

Exercise

After you breathe some deep and open breaths, imagine a beautiful ball of radiant light floating in the air a foot or so in front of your heart. Take a few moments and be fascinated by its beauty. As you look closely, it becomes evident that in the center of this ball is the face of someone who loves you unconditionally. It could be a loved one, a religious figure like Jesus or Buddha, or even a pet.

The closer you look, the more you recognize the unconditional love that is flowing out of that being's eyes toward you. Their eyes twinkle as they radiate a complete acceptance of you exactly as you are. As you gaze into those eyes, allow your heart to open and receive this precious gift. With every in-breath, breathe this love straight into yourself and let a sweet warmth begin to glow in your chest. With each out-breath, send it to every cell of your body. If your struggling mind starts to take over, focus deeply on the radiant love pouring out of that being's eyes.

When you are saturated with this tender warmth, on the next in-breath, breathe the ball of light straight into your heart and see it vibrating and pulsating there. Know that it will always be there. Whenever you are caught in your judging mind, you can bring your attention to your heart area and ask this ball of love to help you open your heart again.

The Voice of Kindness

The third aid in opening a closed heart is a simple method for cultivating an attitude of kindness toward ourselves.

Exercise

Bring into your awareness a person who loves you deeply and imagine what that person would say when you share with her what is happening inside you. A friend of mine once said that she opens the door to her heart again by imagining what Jesus would say about her. If you don't have a connection to a religious figure or a person who loves you unconditionally, imagine what I would say if you shared with me the depth of your closed heart. If what you imagine is kind and understanding, then you would be close to the truth.

This skill — loving ourselves from the inside out — brings us back to the most important kind of relationship we can have with ourselves. I want to stress that it is *okay* to fall in love with ourselves. For even more than we need food, we need to rest in our own hearts. Remember the baby monkeys from chapter 3? We need connection, and we need it most with ourselves. As we learn how to meet ourselves in our own hearts, our actions can come from the wisest part of us. As Jack Kornfield, meditation teacher and author, once wrote, "At the end of life, our questions are very simple: Did I live fully? Did I love well?"[7]

All the love we give to the world stems from the love and acceptance we have for ourselves. It is inside ourselves that we learn how to love our friends, our loved ones, the Earth, and even our enemies. We can't love *out there* if we haven't learned how to love *in here*. We can't stop fighting the world if we haven't yet learned how to stop fighting ourselves and accept ourselves instead.

Yes, it takes courage to cultivate an open heart, and you may need to open it hundreds of times a day. But every time you do, you become a part of the healing of the Earth. Your self-love makes a difference to every human being who lives and will live on this planet. In this opening of your heart, you can let go of focusing on all the hatred and fear that has been gripping human consciousness for thousands of years. Instead, you can shift out of your struggling mind and see it all through the eyes of your heart. As more of us see life this way, humanity will finally fulfill the purpose for which it was brought forth out of Mystery, and life on this planet will know itself at its fullest potential.

Core Ideas

- All people live, to a greater or lesser degree, with the idea that they need to be different from what they are in order to be *okay.*

- Trying to be different from or better than what you are in order to be okay will never work, for it is based on the belief that you are not okay right now.

- We will return to an abiding and ease-filled connection with ourselves and with life only through accepting ourselves as we are.

- You don't have to change anything; you just need to discover the *enoughness* that is you right now.

- There is no better way to learn about self-acceptance than with our compulsions.

- Our perfection lies in our imperfection! The most powerful way to learn about loving ourselves is to acknowledge what we don't do well. We fall in love with ourselves as we learn how to embrace ourselves *as we are* rather than always trying to be what we think we should be.

- Heart energy circumvents the endless game of trying to solve our problems and instead it dissolves them!

- All the desperate wanting behind your compulsive activities is really a longing for tender self-acceptance.

- The most courageous, the most challenging, and also the most healing thing you can do is to fall in love with yourself.

Chapter 9

SKILL THREE:
OPENING TO OUR

Breath

If someone told you that you could magically bring an exhilarating
sense of aliveness, a deep feeling of calm, and a feeling of safety into
your life, would you be interested? Of course you would! The wonderful thing is that you can. There really is something you can do right
now that will bring you all these healing gifts. And you don't have to
purchase anything or go anywhere. All you have to do is breathe, which
brings us to the third skill — Opening to Our Breath.

To open to your breath is to open to yourself. To open to yourself is
to open to life. As we know very well by now, this is what you are truly
hungry for when you are compulsive — a deep and open connection
with yourself and with the present moment of life. Let's explore this
now.

Exercise

Soften your belly and allow a deep breath. Feel the opening of an in-breath — how it lifts your body, making more space within. Now ride the wave of the out-breath, speaking a deep and resonant *ahhhhh*. Allow it to open you to the delicious experience of melting back into just this moment. And again, there is the in-breath, ready to fill you with its healing presence. Take a little time and enjoy each facet of your breath — the opening of the in-breath and the letting go of the out-breath.

Now put the two together by consciously riding the circle of your breath — in-breath turn, out-breath turn — and feel the joy of being fully connected to your breath. If you let go enough you can even feel the experience of being rocked by your breath. Ride this ancient rhythm for a few minutes, giving yourself the gift of simply being. When you are ready, continue reading.

It is amazing when you truly recognize how wonderful it is to breathe consciously in an open and relaxed way. The word *inspiration* literally means "in-breath," for the breath opens us, filling us with more than just oxygen. It brings more spirit into our bodies, our minds, and our emotions. And it is no accident that the sound of a deep and satisfying out-breath is *ahhhhh*, the sound of satisfaction. We express it when we have just finished a great meal, seen a newborn baby, or are trying to let someone know we understand. This sound points us to the release of a full out-breath, a release that allows us to let go and trust ourselves to the living process of life.

The Gifts of Opening to Our Breath

Most likely you have already gone back to more shallow breathing. This type of breathing cuts you off from some of the best things in life: aliveness, connectedness, deep peace, safety, openness, and centeredness. Because you live in a society of shallow breathers, I want to inspire you with all the gifts that open breathing can bring to you. Opening to our breath brings us six core gifts. As you read about these gifts, I invite you to come back over and over again to a deep and slow breath.

A Sense of Aliveness

To breathe is to live. We can survive a month or more without food and a number of days without water, but only a few minutes without breath. And even though our bodies can survive on shallow breathing, they long for deep and open breaths and the aliveness they bring. To breathe fully is to be truly alive. Every cell in our bodies is a little factory that needs raw material to keep working. Much of the food we eat is turned into glucose, a core fuel for our cells. But it takes many molecules of oxygen for every one molecule of glucose for a cell to function efficiently. In other words, the main fuel for our body is oxygen!

When we don't get enough oxygen, the body doesn't work efficiently. (And we wonder why we are tired!) The body is like a wood-burning stove. If we close down the dampers of the stove, stopping the flow of oxygen, the fire will eventually burn out, leaving a lot of ash. But if we open the dampers, the fire will burn brightly. The same is true for our bodies. When we breathe deeply, we bring in more oxygen and our cells glow with aliveness. Often when I thought I was hungry for food, I was truly hungry for some deep breaths.

This vitality doesn't just come from oxygen. Breath contains a healing essence beyond its physical components. Many religions, cultures, and healing systems have cultivated this essence for thousands of years. It is known by a variety of names: *prana* (India), *chi* (China), *ki* (Japan), and *num* (the Kalahari), to name a few. But they are all pointing to the same thing. It is understood that this healing force exists in all forms of matter and is taken up with every breath. Research done with respected tai chi, meditation, and chi kung masters has shown not only that this energy empowers a person but also that it can heal. To breathe normally is to receive some of this energy, but to breathe consciously and freely is to replenish and store this vital substance.

Soften your belly now and allow a deep and slow breath.

Connectedness

Living in shallow breathing supports the notion that each of us is an island unto ourselves. Nothing could be further from the truth. Every time we breathe in, we take in trillions of atoms that were once a part of eagles and butterflies, dinosaurs and stars, slaves and mighty kings. When we breathe out, we send on their way particles that were once an integral part of our bodies, letting them go to a life of infinite adventure. To take a full and complete breath is to open to life on multiple levels, intimately connecting us to the web of existence throughout time and space.

Taking a conscious breath also brings us back to the joy of being in our bodies and reconnects us with the rhythm that is life. The world pulsates with the ebb and flow, the rising and falling of rhythm. It is evident in the tides, the seasons, our hearts, even the peristaltic waves of our intestines. Each of us, as an integral piece of the planet, is joined with the larger rhythms through the pulsations of our bodies, especially our breath. The tides of breath rise and fall every moment of our lives, connecting us to the whole of creation.

Soften your belly now and allow a deep and slow breath.

Deep Peace

Taking an easy, open breath brings deep peace to our whole being. It turns on the parasympathetic nervous system, whose job it is to calm us down. Yet we live mostly with its companion, the sympathetic nervous system. This system says, "Go, go, go; do, do, do!" We live in a society that is addicted to the sympathetic nervous system. We love scary or violent movies. We live at breakneck speeds. We ingest coffee and sugar to stimulate our bodies. (It is probably a good bet to invest in coffee stocks!)

The great rhythm of doing and being, fast and slow, work and rest is broken by our love affair with speed. This speed always takes us away from ourselves, leaving us more vulnerable to the ravages of compulsion. This is one of the main reasons that we are usually more inclined to be compulsive at the end of the day. We have spent our time running as fast as we can and moving farther and farther from ourselves, and to stop feels uncomfortable at first. To breathe deeply turns on the calming part of our nervous system. This brings us back to ourselves, to sanity and to calm, even in the middle of a busy day.

Soften your belly now and allow a deep and slow breath.

Sanctuary

The breath is a sanctuary that is available to us no matter where we are or what is happening in our lives. Whenever my mind is restless, instead of searching for peace *out there* in another mouthful of food or in getting things under control or in some other heart-numbing activity, I now have a place where my attention can return — the rising and falling of my breath. It brings me back into my body, into the here and now and into the wellspring of wisdom and support within.

Every morning and for a number of times throughout the day, I allow my attention to rest in this ancient rhythm. Because I have become friends with my breath, I actually feel like the great Mother of Life is rocking me in a cradle. Those moments are like minivacations that allow my mind to quiet down and insight to flood my awareness.

Soften your belly now and allow a deep and slow breath.

Dissolving Old Patterns

Opening to our breath also minimizes the deepest pains of human life. We all have a tendency to tighten down around physical pain. When we do, it only makes the pain worse. Imagine somebody squeezing your hand until it hurts and then, when you say it hurts, they squeeze it more. We do this to ourselves with headaches, backaches, injuries; we even do it when we're at the dentist. Our muscles tighten down around the pain. We can reverse the process by breathing into the experience, allowing our breath to expand into it, much like blowing up a balloon. It not only frees up the cramping, it also opens space for the blood vessels to bring the necessary ingredients for healing.

We can breathe into our emotions as well. Over and over, I have watched people in the throes of a deep emotion react to what they are experiencing and then react to their reaction. When I invite them to bring their attention to the part in their body that has tightened because of the emotion and then to breathe into the sensations that are there, most people are amazed at how this lightens the experience.

When you are being overtaken by an emotion — whether it is anger, fear, sadness, or a variation of one of those — taking a few deep breaths focused on the physical sensations of that emotion can transform your experience. What we fail to see is that emotions are amplified when we resist them. When we participate with them instead — and one of the simplest and most profound ways of doing that is through breathing into them — many of them become like clouds moving through us rather than a storm that "rains on our parade." I call this the Balloon Breath, and it is one of the most powerful tools we have to dissolve the old patterns within us that fuel our compulsions. I invite you to try it:

Exercise

After you take a few deep breaths, bring your attention into your breath, feeling it from the inside. Feel how the in-breath expands and opens your body and how the out-breath carries with it a sense of letting go. Now find a tight spot in your body and imagine that your breath is a balloon that you are blowing up inside you, right at the experience of tightness. On every in-breath, pull air into the balloon, allowing it to gently push against the tension you find there. Then let go on the out-breath, saying out loud a long and slow *ahhhhh*. Do this for a number of breaths, each time expanding a little bit more the area of tension. Your tension will respond to the gentle but opening pressure of the breath.

Soften your belly now and allow a deep and slow breath.

Centeredness

Taking an open breath also brings the center of gravity down into your body, tapping you into the wellspring of wisdom in the belly — an amazingly powerful and healing place to live from. Just as an umbilical cord connected us to our mother when we were in the womb, an energy umbilical cord in our belly connects us to the wellspring within us that is sourced from the wisdom at the heart of life.

When we were young, we were grounded in our bellies, and this energy umbilical cord still pulsated with vitality. This is one of the reasons we were able to be so alive in our play. Rooted in the nourishing soil of our bellies, we could whirl and twirl, leap and dance with a sense of balance that is lost to most adults. It is also why, in our younger years, we were so resilient in the face of deep emotions.

Can you imagine twirling and tumbling like you did when you were a child? As adults, we usually keep our center of gravity in our heads with shallow breathing. Having lost the sense of balance that comes from being connected to our bellies, we are like top-heavy trees, vulnerable to the storms of our lives and the unconscious illusion that we can take care of ourselves through our compulsions. Cultivating an open breath takes us back into the safety of being connected to our bellies and all the spontaneity and trust that lives there.

To watch somebody who naturally breathes from the belly is a thing of beauty. Whether it is a postman or an accomplished ballerina, when someone is connected to her belly through her breath, her movements are wondrous to behold. We recognize in her an alive connectedness that touches us to the core.

Soften your belly now and allow a deep and slow breath.

As you can now see, to give ourselves the gift of a full and open breath is one of the most healing things we can do, for healing is about opening what has been closed, softening what has been hardened. The wonderful thing about breath is that it heals us on all levels of our being — physical, emotional, mental, spiritual. I can't describe how much I love a deep breath that comes from my belly. It reminds me of the kind of joy I know when I am laughing so hard I almost pee in my pants. It also reminds me of lying under the stars with nothing to separate me from deep reverence for life. It can even bring back the essence of those moments when I was looking into my lover's eyes, giving and receiving love with every cell of my being. In all these experiences, my belly was soft, my breath was free, and I was animated from my core. As we learn how to connect with our breath again, it can become both our teacher and our healer, taking us back into what we are truly hungry for — intimate, alive, and loving connection with ourselves and with life.

Soften your belly now and allow a deep and slow breath.

Breathing through Our Compulsions

As we become more intimate with our breath, not only does it bring us all the gifts we have explored, it also assumes the role of a wise and benevolent teacher. It is full of valuable information that can show us how to relate to a wave of compulsion rather than becoming lost in it.

From our very first breath until our last, our lives are a continuous river of breathing in which the experiences of life flow along. When we first learned to ride a tricycle, this river was breathing us. When we laughed and when we cried it was breathing us. Every time we were swimming, showering, shopping, kissing, singing, and sleeping it was breathing us. Every breath has been different, influenced not only by the needs of our body but also by our thoughts and emotions. It is fast when we are excited and slow when we are resting. It can be shallow when we are angry and deeper when we are at peace.

If we watch the ever-changing nature of breath, it will tell us how close or far away we are from ourselves. Whenever we are caught in our heads, with its continuous addiction to control, we tighten our bellies and breathe more shallowly. This contraction indicates that we are cut off from the nourishment of being connected to ourselves and thus are vulnerable to being compulsive. As we learn how to be attuned to breath, it can point out to us very early in a wave of compulsion that we are in need of connection. As we become more in tune with ourselves, it can alert us even before the wave begins.

As we learn how to breathe down into our bellies again, our open breathing awakens our wellspring of deep knowing. In this awakening, we find that it becomes easier and easier to make wise and skillful choices, even in the face of the urge to be compulsive. For, as we discussed in chapter 4, our empowered no is a part of the wellspring of wisdom in our bellies. At the heart of this type of no lies a yes to life — a yes to balance, skillful living, and peace.

Notice what your breath is doing right now. Are you holding onto it or letting it freely rise and fall? I first became aware of how much I held my breath while watching cartoons with my children. Now, as far as I can see, watching TV is usually not life threatening. But while watching the Road Runner approaching a cliff with Wily Coyote hot on his trail, I saw that I had pulled up and contracted my whole body, especially the right side, and was hardly breathing at all.

I had had enough contact at this point with the joys of open breathing that I was curious about this old pattern of contraction. As I began to watch my breath throughout the day, to my amazement the only time I experienced an open breath was early in the morning when I was by myself and felt completely safe. As the day wore on, my breathing usually got tighter and my connection with myself became dimmer, making me more vulnerable to my compulsion.

I wanted to stay in contact with myself, nourished by this connection for more than an hour or two in the morning, and my breath became an exquisite biofeedback system. It showed me when I was tightening down and turning away from myself again. I began to retrain this ancient response by softening my body and taking a deep breath whenever I noticed how contracted I had become. This brought my attention out of the narrowness of my mind and into the spaciousness of my body. At the beginning, I could only do this when I was sitting still. Slowly I became able to breathe back into myself as I moved throughout my day.

As I became more receptive to the experience of my breath (and the joy of an open one), I saw that contraction was always present when I was caught up in a wave of compulsion. At first I couldn't do anything except watch. The grip my struggling mind had on my breath was too strong. But as I played with my breath when my compulsions were quiet, I began to feel the profound satisfaction of my breath going all the way down to my belly. It not only felt right, but I could see that a deep hunger inside me was satisfied when I allowed my breath to be that open — the hunger for being connected to myself.

It took me a while to learn that when the hunger of compulsion would appear, rather than heading down the ever-tightening spiral of reaction, I could feed it with a few deep breaths. These breaths reconnected me with myself, and often the wave would pass through, leaving hardly a ripple. Other times, when my compulsion needed more than just a few breaths to feed it, opening to my breath put me in contact with exactly what I was experiencing. Usually it was something uncomfortable that was fueling the compulsion. Through this contact, I took back my power. When I turned toward the experience, using my breath to open to exactly what was going on rather than being devoured by the experience (the main fear of the mind), I could now recognize what was happening.

In this recognition, I had the choice either to be present with what I was experiencing, allowing my undivided attention to transform these tight places within me back into the free-flowing energy they came from, or to close down and run away again. All my life I had been running, and when I first started being present for myself when I was compulsive, I still ran sometimes. But shallow breathing was always there to remind me that running away just made the experience worse.

Breathing into Our Wellspring of Wisdom

Opening to our breath also puts us in contact with a source of Intelligence that, thankfully, is much smarter than anything we can figure out on our own. If we watch carefully, we will see that whenever a wave of compulsion knocks us over, it feels like we are David facing Goliath and that there is no help for miles around. Yet nothing could be further from the truth. In our bodies lies our wellspring of wisdom that is connected to the very Intelligence that gave us life in the first place. This Intelligence is waiting to help us with our compulsions.

We can begin to understand the depth of wisdom within our bodies by looking at the intricate creativity it took to bring forth human beings in the first place. It is astounding that life has been able to bring the light of the universe into the living, breathing being that is you, a person who can see and touch and hear and celebrate the awesome wonder of life. We could say that each of us is light that has learned how to see, hear, taste, touch, and describe itself. Our limited minds can't even begin to comprehend this, let alone explain it. Nonetheless, we get all the benefits from the imaginative inventiveness of life — we get to be alive!

Not only are you a recipient of this Intelligence, you *are* a field of Intelligence. It resides inside every cell of your body and is most evident in the ribbon of information called DNA. This is the blueprint that makes you *you*. Each cell is less than 1/1,000 of an inch across, and yet it contains enough information to fill one thousand books with six hundred pages each! If you uncoiled the ribbons of DNA from all the cells of your body and placed them end on end, they would stretch to the moon — which is more than two hundred and thirty thousand miles away — and back one hundred thousand times!

Before you go on to the next sentence, let that sink in. I think we can safely say that the Intelligence that orchestrates our bodies is greater than all the knowledge that human beings have ever gathered. Not only does this Intelligence operate inside individual cells, but when these cells come together into communities called bodies (or organisms), it also orchestrates a complexity of processes that boggles the mind. Imagine driving a car, talking on a cell phone, and trying to listen to directions from a passenger. This is almost impossible to do, and yet it is only three tasks. Your body administers zillions of tasks every moment of your life. There are so many that it is impossible to comprehend. And yet your body hardly ever misses a beat.

As humanity has crawled up into the attic of our minds, we have learned how to rely on our own resources, cutting ourselves off from the vast sea of Intelligence that is life and the wisdom and support that are always with us. Feel your body, as you are reading this book. You will find myriad sensations — pressure, heat, itches, and pain. If you pay deep attention, encompassing all those is a vibration, an aliveness. That is the field of Intelligence.

This Intelligence is often given the name God, and then all sorts of definitions and rules spring up around it. In a workshop I attended, author Stephen Levine once said, "I can use the word God because I have absolutely no idea what it means, but there is nowhere that I see it not!" Contrary to many popular religious beliefs, contact with this Intelligence does not happen in some far-off place (usually after you die), only granted if you have lived your life "right." The doorway to immediate and intimate contact with this Intelligence is inside you right now.

One of the many gifts that compulsions provide is that they won't let us off the hook until we stop trying to live our lives all by ourselves. Compulsions are here to invite, cajole, push, and prod us back into our bodies and into recognition and connection with this Intelligence. We will explore how to ask for help from the wellspring of wisdom within us in chapter 12. Until then, know that opening to our breath brings us back into our bodies, making us receptive to the awesome field of Intelligence that resides there. This Intelligence will guide us in listening for what we truly need at any given moment of our life — not for what we want, but what we need.

Practices for Nourishing Ourselves with Breath

To be in contact with our breath is a wondrous thing. As we have been exploring, deep and open breathing brings a vitality and a calmness into our bodies that is positively delicious. It also nourishes the deep hunger we have for an intimate relationship with ourselves. As we cultivate an awareness of what our breath is doing, it also becomes our friend, signaling when we are disconnecting from ourselves. The breath can then be used as a great healer, transforming our formerly frozen feelings into the joy of flowing energy. Yet most of us aren't even aware of the healing rhythm of our breath that is happening right under (and through!) our noses. Breathing unconsciously and shallowly, we are cut off from the friendship of our breath.

The most important thing we can do to access the joy of alive and open breathing is simply to notice how much we hold our breath. And, in some ways, that is enough. We can't force ourselves to breathe openly again. That kind of struggle is exactly what caused us to hold our breath in the first place. But we can become curious not only about how much we hold our breath but also about how wonderful it feels when we don't. That noticing begins to seed a process whereby we *want* to be in contact with our natural breath rather than feeling that we *have to* make our breath be different from what it is.

From this longing to know free breathing again, you can begin to cultivate your deep natural breath. I invite you to play with it right now as you are reading.

Exercise

The next time you breathe out, when you come to what you think is the end of your out-breath, keep on breathing out, slightly pulling in around the region of your belly button. When you do this, you will discover that a lot more air is left in your lungs and this slight pressure can gently push it out.

When you come to the completion of the out-breath, let your belly go and feel the in-breath come flooding in, lifting and opening your body. As the in-breath turns again into an out-breath, watch how you can let go of much more air when you include your belly. Make this a gentle push. Don't force it. When you come to the end of the out-breath feel the joy of softening your belly, making space for the in-breath. The more space you make in your lungs through a full out-breath, the deeper your in-breath will be. Keep breathing deeply as you are reading, getting a sense of what it is like when you involve your belly again in your breathing.

This is the art of full and open breathing, the kind of breathing that nourishes you from the inside out. The key to this kind of breath is to focus on the exhalation. At first it may feel a little awkward, a little like trying to rub your tummy and pat your head at the same time. But the body knows how to breathe this way, and with a little bit of coaching your natural breath can begin to make itself known again. You can then let go of consciously pulling in your belly as you are breathing out, for the body will deeply exhale on its own.

You aren't trying to make the breath stay in the belly — that would just be more struggle. But when you take a moment to consciously cultivate a deep and full breath, you change your breathing from shallow to open and from tight to free. You can then remember the joy of open breathing, and in that remembering become more attuned to when you are again holding your breath.

Exercise

Notice your breath again. It has probably left your belly and is again in the upper part of your chest. Don't try to change it. Just notice how different this breath is from the open breathing you played with a few minutes ago. Stay with your shallow breathing, becoming familiar with how it feels. It is important to know both extremes of breath — the open, free breath and the shallow, contracted breath.

When we practice full and open breathing we bring a center of vitality, safety, and creativity into our lives. Familiarity with shallow breathing attunes your awareness so that when you are holding your breath again, that familiarity will wake you up, indicating that something needs your attention. With this familiarity, you can begin to use your breath to signal yourself when you are heading down the path to compulsion.

To attune yourself to the nourishment of an open breath and to use the shallow breath as a signal that you are disconnecting from yourself, it is helpful simply to pay attention to your breath at certain times every day. I do this every morning. For a few minutes, I breathe the deep and open breath that we explored earlier. This always quiets my mind and brings a sense of vitality to my body. I then allow my breath to be exactly as it wants to be, and I bring my attention to the experience. To spend even a few minutes a day in curiosity about the breath creates a relationship with this wise and wondrous teacher, a relationship that will guide you in healing and being healed by your compulsion.

It is also helpful to pause throughout the day and simply take one full breath. If it moves into a number of deep breaths that's great, but just one will do wonders for your life. Because it is so easy to forget to breathe open breaths, try to connect a deep breath to something that you do repeatedly throughout the day, giving yourself these nourishing moments where you are returning to yourself. I do this every time I wash my hands. All our moments of waiting — at the doctor's office, in rush-hour traffic, or in all the lines we stand in — can become moments when we cultivate a deep and open breath.

Another favorite breathing exercise of mine is to imagine on my out-breath that I have roots growing out of the bottom of my feet and down into the earth. As I become as grounded as a tree, on my in-breaths I imagine the deep nourishment of the earth filling me with its presence as I send my roots ever deeper on my out-breaths. This is wonderful to do while waiting for an elevator, standing on your porch in the early morning, cooking dinner, and so on. It cultivates a centered strength that is deeply grounding and nourishing.

It is very important not to make either open breathing or paying attention to your breath into *shoulds*, engaging in the same struggling mind that created compulsions in the first place. These words are an invitation, and for some of you that will be enough. If you don't force these practices, they will become seeds that will grow into full and open breathing in your own time and in your own way. Trust where you are. At the same time, trust that a free and open breath is your destiny, for it is an essential component of a deep and nourishing connection with yourself and with life.

Soften your belly now and allow a deep and slow breath.

Core Ideas

- Open breathing is a sanctuary that is available to us no matter where we are or what is happening in our lives.

- Open breathing brings the center of gravity down into your body, tapping you into the wellspring of wisdom in the belly.

- Opening to our breath lessens the deepest pains of human life. This is most evident on the physical level, but it also works like magic on our emotions.

- When compulsions appear, rather than heading down the ever-tightening spiral of reaction, just take a few deep breaths.

- Pause throughout the day and simply take one full breath. If it moves into a number of deep breaths that's great, but just one will do wonders for your life.

- Every time that you pause for just a moment, take a breath, and check in with yourself, you take another step along the path of healing.

Chapter 10

SKILL FOUR:
COMING HOME TO
Ourselves

I f we watch ourselves closely when we are compulsive, we'll realize not only that we are trying to get away from an uncomfortable sensation or feeling, but also that we are trying to move toward the experience of feeling good again. Take, for example, a difficult day at work when your boss yells at you and then your co-workers go out to lunch without asking you along. For many of us, deep and uncomfortable feelings would build throughout the day until, without a thought, we find ourselves buying a six-pack even though we have sworn off alcohol. Or we discover in our laps enough food for three people after we have exited the drive-through.

As we plunge into overeating, overdrinking, overshopping, more unconscious sex, or another cigarette, for a few moments the tension eases and everything seems okay. That hazy glow that comes after a couple of beers or the safe feeling that comes from having a full stomach seems to take us out of the pain and back into ease again — that is, until the consequences of our actions and the ensuing self-judgment rear their ugly heads. We pay such a heavy price for taking care of ourselves this way, a price that becomes higher and higher the older we get. As we know by now, it is never our compulsions that we are truly longing for. What we truly long for is the ability to be present with ourselves and with our lives. We make this kind of connection by cultivating the power of simply *being*. Let me give you an example. I was writing the other day, sitting on the couch in the room I use for counseling, when suddenly I became aware of warmth on my foot. As I looked up, there was the morning sun, caressing my leg. Joy burst forth from deep within me as the past and the future faded away and all that was left was the sun on my leg, a deep sense of delight coursing through my body, and a keen appreciation for the gift of life. In those moments, I was *here*, fully present for myself and for my life. Oh, the joy of simply being!

An important element of coming home to ourselves is relearning the joy of simply being. Underneath all our busyness, what we truly long for is to find fulfillment in the "enoughness" of this moment. Even though it is one of the most profound things a human being can do, most of us have forgotten how. Our minds are usually planning what is going to happen, rehashing what did happen, and struggling with everything in between. We love to acquire and do, fix and achieve, attain and figure out. There is nothing wrong with these activities except that when they become our primary mode of existence, they cut us off from the astounding healing of simply *being*. This makes us vulnerable to the seduction of compulsions. But no compulsion can ever quench our longing to be truly awake to life, experiencing the joy of being at home with ourselves and with our lives. And that is what this chapter will explore: the fourth skill, Coming Home to Ourselves.

When we relearn how to simply *be*, we begin to discover moments, like the one I experienced with the sun on my leg, in which our minds, our bodies, and our hearts are all in the same place at the same time. These moments hold the power to heal us to our core. The more we cultivate them, the more connected we become. The more connected we become, the more we live from the wellspring within that holds all the clarity, peace, wisdom, and joy that we long for. We then learn how to use our doing, fixing, achieving mind when we need it, allowing it to fade into the background again as we discover the truth and the beauty of life as it is, right here and right now.

Beliefs that Keep Us from Being

Perhaps these words strike a chord deep within you. On some level we all recognize that we are not connected to ourselves and our lives, and yet we are afraid of the kind of connection I am talking about. *We are afraid of simply being!* Try to live a day without your favorite distraction — reading, talking, or watching TV. Instead, simply open to life. If you do this, you will see what I am talking about. You will probably get anxious, frustrated, bored, or depressed. You will be caught in your mind, unable to simply *be*.

And yet in *being*, all the wonders of this marvelous adventure reveal themselves. Gilda Radner, the comedian who died of ovarian cancer, once said that if it weren't for the downside of cancer (possible death), everybody should experience it because it teaches us how to deeply appreciate and open to the miracle of existence. She is not the only one who discovered this truth. Many people living with a terminal diagnosis describe it as one of the most alive times of their lives.

Why, when being is so wonderful, do we insist on staying stuck in the attics of our minds? We are not made to live in the attic, which so quickly becomes a prison instead of the safe haven we initially sought. It is our destiny to know the full house of our being, and all the joy, trust, and peace that reside there. To open the door to the rest of the house again, we need to look at four core beliefs we took on while stuck up in the attic, beliefs that keep us locked away from the healing of simply being.

It Is Not Safe to Open to Life Again

Life is for us. Our everyday experiences aren't just a series of disconnected events in which it sometimes seems that the Intelligence in charge of it all has fallen asleep on the job. In fact, the exact opposite is true. There is a powerful and benevolent intent behind absolutely everything that happens in our lives. Life wants us to awaken into its full presence even more than we do, and it is giving us all the experiences we need to relearn the safety and the exhilaration of being open to our lives.

So the first belief we need to dismantle to open the door to *being* is that it is not safe to open to life. For most of us, this was true when we were growing up. We didn't have the skills or the wisdom to meet life as it was. But we are not children anymore, and to stay caught in the narrow room of the intellect has become unsafe. All the stories in our heads keep us in the past and in the future, and we are rarely present and alert to what is happening right now. To live in our heads is like walking along the edge of a cliff with a blindfold on. If that isn't unsafe, I don't know what is!

In addition, the stories in our heads tell us that they are keeping us safe through control. But if we watch closely, we will see that the lions and tigers and bears of our lives live mostly in the exact place we have gone when trying to hide from life — in the attic of the mind. In the ongoing conversation we have with ourselves all day long we find the lions of our hatreds and fears, the tigers of our compulsions, and the bears of our despair. And since there is very little space up there, it is very easy to stay in reaction, tumbling from one struggle to another, completely cut off from life. We need to understand that cultivating being is not about being powerless. It is not about being out of control. Even though at first glance being seems like just rolling over and passively letting life do with us as it will, it is the exact opposite. Cultivating being puts us in a very active place where we are passionately alert, listening and learning from every experience we are given. Something happens when we stay this open and passionately listen. We begin to realize that life is speaking to us all the time. It gives us the clues that will take us out of our reactive mind and back into the joy of being truly connected to life. Remember those connect-the-dot puzzles from childhood where, when we followed the numbers with our pencil, the picture became clear? That is very similar to the experience of coming home to ourselves. As we learn how to listen, really listen, to whatever we are being given, it begins to make sense.

To trust our journey at that level, we need to look at our relationship with pain, for this is why we closed off in the first place. It hurts to be alive. It hurts to stub your toe, to be rejected, to lose a loved one. When we were young, the pains of our lives were amplified dramatically. Time is different for a child. Five minutes felt like an hour, an hour like a day, and a day like a week. The only skill for coping with pain that we learned was to resist it. So we held our breath and tightened our muscles, hiding feelings deep in our bodies and retreating to our minds. For a while that worked, but that didn't mean that whatever we were trying to run away from would simply vanish. In fact, the opposite was true. Pain fermented inside us, turning into pure fuel for our compulsions and exploding all over our lives in the most unpleasant ways.

It took me a long time to see that when I resist pain, whether it is physical, mental, or emotional, it always gets worse. As a wise teacher once said, "Pain is a given in human experience. Suffering is our resistance to our pain." We can understand what this means when we see that life is a dance of duality. One day we feel clear as a bell, and the next day confusion reigns. One morning we get up and our body feels light and alive. The next morning we don't know how we can make it through the day. For a time, our new relationship is easy and full of fun. Then it turns into a war that seems to have no origin. That is what life is like. One day is very stormy, and then we wake up to sunshine the next day.

When we try to have only the pleasant stuff, it all turns into a struggle. When we try to run away from the pains of our lives, we also cut ourselves off from our joy. We can't have one without the other. It also took me a while to discover that if I open to my pain in curiosity, I bring it out of the shadows into the light where I can work with it in kind and skillful ways. Pain is so much more workable when we stay open to it. The easiest place to see this truth is in your body. Even physical therapists and doctors now know that if you teach a person how to open around their pain, it not only lessens, it also hastens the time of healing.

This has certainly been true in my body. I have had much physical pain in my life, and for years all I did was resist it. I took pills. I overate. I tried to distract myself in every way, and my pain stayed stuck to me like glue. When I learned how to open to it and acknowledge it, it became much more bearable, and I discovered that right in the heart of the pain was all the wisdom needed to bring it back into balance. Not only did this technique work with my physical pain, but it also did wonders with all the emotional pain that I had run from my whole life. I have also seen it work like magic with friends, clients, and loved ones. When they share with me the depth of their suffering, they are usually holding their breath, tightening their bodies, and their minds are spinning out of control.

By inviting them to go toward the experience rather than turning away, I take them into their bodies, asking them to name and then experience what is going on. Invariably they take a big breath, discovering that it isn't as scary as they thought, and whatever is happening becomes workable again. Keep in mind that just taking a few deep breaths when you are in pain, whether it is physical, mental, or emotional, and softening your belly can lessen the pain. As you open, you can then discover that, rather than being your enemy, your pain is a wise and benevolent teacher, revealing to you the place where you are caught in reaction. If you listen, it will show you the way beyond the struggles of your mind.

This is why I call my pain my noble adversary. As I grappled with the great challenges of my pains, they sharpened my attention, opened my heart, and taught me how to truly listen. They invited me to be open to my own journey — to the pleasant and the unpleasant, the joys and the sorrows. They then showed me that when I can meet myself as I am and open to my life exactly as it is, the joy that is my birthright would make itself known. Not only is it safe to open to life, but it is only in opening to whatever is right here, right now that we will discover the connection and the peace that we long for. Let us explore the safety of opening in the following exercise:

Exercise

Close your eyes and take some deep breaths. Every time you breathe out, let go. Let go of the tension in your neck, your shoulder blades, your belly, and even your feet. Let it all go and amplify this letting go by saying *ahhhhh*. Now let go of all your thoughts about the past and the future, and ground your attention in your immediate experience. Feel warmth and coolness, along with the pulsating and vibrating that is your body.

As you settle into your body, feel yourself sitting. Feel the pressure on your legs, your buttocks, and your back. When you make contact with the experience of sitting, with every out-breath, melt into whatever you are sitting on and let it hold you. If it is hard to make this shift of perception from sitting "on top of" to being held, imagine the support beneath you all of a sudden evaporating. You would fall to the floor! So it is true that you are sitting on top of something, but you are also being held. For these few moments, let go of sitting "on top of" and allow yourself to be held.

Now expand your awareness. Whatever you are sitting on is being held by the floor beneath it. And the floor is being held by the foundation and the foundation by the Earth. Now, what is the Earth being held by? Allow your awareness to expand so that you can imagine looking down through the floor, the foundation, the crust of the Earth, and even the center of the Earth. Keep on going, and as your awareness pops out on the other side of the Earth, you see with astonishment that the Earth is being held by space. It isn't stuck on a stick or hung by a string. It allows itself to be held by nothing more substantial than space. And yet it is fully supported.

Now bring your awareness back to yourself sitting here. Recognize that as you sit, you too are being held by the same space that is holding the Earth. Allow yourself to trust life enough for this moment that you see that wherever you are, whatever is happening, you are being held by life.

My Body Is Not My Friend

Since *being* is about making immediate contact with ourselves and with life, it means we have to be in our bodies. But most of us don't live there. We have been hijacked by the style of thinking that says the body is just a vehicle for maneuvering through our lives. We have been brainwashed into riding around inside of a mind that sits on top of a body, never aware that what we truly long for is to live in our bodies again.

Irish novelist James Joyce wrote this wonderful line: "Mr. Duffy lives a short distance from his body!"[1] When we were young, we were naturally in contact with how delicious it was to have a body. We lived inside our bodies, inside ourselves, and we were in contact with our inner wellspring. Over time we learned that it wasn't safe or accepted by the adults around us to be this open and alive. We retreated to the attic of our minds (which is for most of us a very long distance from our bodies!) and tightened our muscles, discovering that we rarely, if ever, feel at ease with ourselves, at home in our bodies.

Lost in the ivory towers of our intellects, we are almost completely out of touch with our bodies, and at the same time we are obsessed with their appearance. The average model is five feet eleven inches tall and weighs 110 pounds, and we try to emulate them! Who weighs that little when they are that tall? Only people in countries that are facing starvation — and models. Not only do we judge our bodily appearances, we also load much of our self-hate onto them. Think of all the self-destructive behaviors that are acted out on the body: overloading it with food, drugs, and alcohol; biting our fingernails; engaging in meaningless sex; picking our skin; expecting the body to work endless hours fueled only by coffee, sugar, and high-fat foods.

Here is this wondrous creation that we have been given, which we have learned to disregard and disrespect. From Christian theologians such as St. Augustine, who was caught in his own struggling mind, and our misinterpretation of the writings of the Apostle Paul, we bought into the belief that the body and its emotions, needs, and feelings were beneath the world of the spirit. From Plato came the idea that "we must avoid as much as we can all contact and association with the body, except when they are absolutely necessary."[2]

It wasn't only religion and philosophy that cut us off from our bodies; science didn't help either. It divided life into parts, missing the interconnectedness of it all. As science explored the various parts of the body, it missed the deep intelligence of the body as a whole. In scientists' urge to divide in order to understand, they reduced all of life to a mechanistic universe made up of inert atoms, separate unto themselves, with no spark of spirit within them.

Yet no depiction could be more inaccurate. Our bodies are a gift from life. They are nothing less than magnificent, no matter what shape, size, color, or age. They are also an unfolding sea of creativity that is more intelligent, more ancient, and more alive than we can possibly imagine. Even those so-called static building blocks of life called atoms are pulsating with energy. If you blew up an atom to the size of a baseball field, the nucleus would be just a grain of sand out by the pitcher's mound, and the electrons would be dancing beyond the outer edge of the field. What fills up the rest of the space? Nothing less than vibrating, pulsating, creative waves and particles of light. This is not just fanciful thinking; it is the conclusion of many of our leading-edge scientists.

Think about it: you are nothing less than a field of creative light! The more you are present in your body, the more it shines. Matthew Fox, in his book *Sins of the Spirit, Blessings of the Flesh,* reported that if we were able to harness all the light in one human being, we could turn on all of the floodlights it takes to light a major league baseball field and keep them lit for three hours.[3] When we inhabit our own bodies, in contact with all that light, we receive two gifts: the joy of being alive and a sense of deep knowing.

It is so delicious to be *in* our bodies. The body is a river of free-flowing aliveness that nourishes us to our core. This energy wants to leap and soar, being as expressive as the sun and as still as a clear mountain pool, infusing us with radiance. We are starved for the glow of being! Think of the eyes of someone in love. They are glowing because of their inner light. We often think of great spiritual leaders with halos around their heads. This is how we symbolize the truth that their light field has been turned up full volume. We can know this glow too as we make friends with our bodies again.

When we connect with our own joy, we enter the web of joy that permeates everything. Everywhere we look life celebrates the joy of existence — the beauty in the unfolding of a flower, the dance of dandelion seeds on the wind, the purr of a cat, or the music of a waterfall. *Joy is nothing less than the energy of life celebrating itself freely.* Sit quietly and watch a tree long enough that you can begin to feel it stretching its branches out to the sun. You can feel this propensity for joy in the sound of water cascading across rocks and in the play of the wind in the leaves. And you are an integral part of this unfolding of joy that is life!

Inhabiting our bodies also brings us in contact with our own deep knowing. When we begin to listen, to really listen to our bodies, we discover that they are constantly speaking to us, giving us the clues to our healing. We also discover that as we listen, we can hear more easily the deep wisdom within us. I discovered this while doing massage many years ago. I had learned numerous techniques and was busily applying what I thought I should be doing. My massages were good, but not great. I then began to notice that some massages were more alive than others. I realized that with the clients who were having a "wow" kind of experience, I was massaging from a different place. Rather than thinking about what I should be doing, *I was listening to what my own body was asking for!* My inner radar was telling me exactly what was appropriate for the person to whom I was giving a massage. And the more I listened, the more people left feeling truly connected to themselves.

I then began to apply this in other aspects of my life, especially with my children. I would listen in my body for the appropriate words or actions in any given situation. When I spoke from this place, a place that felt *right* inside me, it always brought clarity and lessened dramatically the normal resistance of teenagers. They respected what I said when they recognized that I was speaking from this clear place.

To help you become more at home in your body, I offer below a powerful meditation. It can stand on its own, or you can add it at the beginning of your daily Returning Practice. This meditation opens up the pockets of tension in your body so that your energy can flow freely:

Exercise

After you read through this exercise, close your eyes, take a few deep breaths, and let go as deeply as you can on each out-breath. Then allow your breath to be as it wants. As you settle into its rhythm, feel your body. It is a constantly changing river of sensation, different right now than it ever has been. Simply feel what it is experiencing in this moment.

Now, using your attention like a flashlight, bring it to the top of your head. As you let it rest there, the sensations in your head will reveal themselves, just like a Polaroid picture developing. If the sensations are hazy, ask yourself, "How do I even know there is a head there?" This invites the mind to be curious, exploring what is there. Stay there for at least thirty seconds — more if it is an area that intrigues you today.

Then bring your attention to your face and see what is happening there. Again, use your attention like a flashlight. There are numerous sensations — tickles, warmth, pressure, moisture. Slowly work your way around your face just as if you were exploring a new country. When you come to your lips, wet them with your tongue and see what happens. Then draw your attention inside your mouth and recognize your tongue. Allow it to explore all the varied surfaces in your mouth.

Now move down into your throat. As you settle in, what do you discover there? Is there tightness? If so, is it more on the right or on the left? Go around to the back of your neck and see what is there. Again, whenever you move your attention, let it settle in the new spot for a few moments. Rather than trying to find the sensations, allow them to reveal themselves to you.

There is no set pattern to this meditation. If it intrigues you, explore both your arms and hands with your curiosity. Or maybe your back interests you today. Wherever you go, notice if you have any areas that you like more than others and any areas that you are resistant to being with. If you find an area with a lot of tension, know that you have been resisting whatever is there.

One of the very powerful areas to make contact with is your belly. We hold a lot of tension in the belly, both on the surface and deep within. There is also a tremendous wellspring of aliveness there, and as you pay attention, this wellspring will reveal itself.

Be sure to explore the whole pelvic floor too, for as it opens, energy can cascade down your legs, grounding you right here and now. As you explore your legs, see if any tension blocks this energy. As you make contact with your feet, check in with one first, exploring it as intimately as you can, and then go to the other. Notice both the similarities and the differences in sensations. When you are done, take your attention back to your whole body and notice how it has changed now that you have spent intimate time with it.

This is a wonderful gift to give yourself — the gift of being fully present with your body. The miracle of your body is being touched by the healing power of your attention. You can take two minutes to do this meditation, just exploring your face, or you can take an hour, exploring every nook and cranny of your body. You can also explore the more surface sensations, or you can go deep inside, feeling the rhythm of your breath from inside your chest and the pulse of your heart throughout your body. Know that every time you check in with yourself this way, you are taking another step into living *in* your body, connected to the river of aliveness that you are.

My Feelings Will Overwhelm Me

The wondrous thing is that when we cultivate *being*, especially being present for ourselves, the feelings we have run from our whole lives lose their power over us. "No. No," says the controlling mind. "If I stop running and become present, my anger, my sadness, or my fear will overwhelm me." At first glance this does seem true. Remember a time when you finally could not keep up the pace of your "doing" life and, rather than settling down into relaxation and fun, all sorts of heavy states, including that of your compulsion, took over.

But look at the same experience with the understanding that these feelings wanted to be recognized and then let go of, and you just didn't know how to do this. As you slow down, rather than trying to get away from what you are experiencing, you become willing to be present for yourself as you are. Of course the feelings you have been ignoring begin to surface, and rather than running away, you meet them with deep compassion and understanding, and you feel empowered to your core. These feelings, rather than taking over your life, have now been brought into the light of your consciousness where they can be met with understanding and transformed with compassion.

At the beginning, as we are learning the skills of engaging rather than managing, this can be a bit of a bumpy ride. We may only be able to meet what we are experiencing for a moment or two before we fall into reaction — before we go from "Ah, this is fear" to "I am so afraid." But just one moment of meeting our feelings as they are is much more powerful than a million moments of thinking that we *are* the feelings and thus getting lost inside them. We will explore how to meet and let go of our feelings in part 4. Until then, know that turning toward a feeling and meeting it with your attention lessens the power it has over you.

Cultivating Being Is Selfish

Most of us believe that to spend time with ourselves — to cultivate *being* — is inherently selfish. This idea holds great power in our society, pressuring us to prove that we are not just standing around taking up space and, heaven forbid, enjoying ourselves. Most people are so terrified of being labeled selfish that they run around like chickens with their heads cut off trying to prove their worth. Even with all that doing, they still carry secret fears deep inside that they are selfish and self-absorbed. In this disconnection, their actions become reactions rather than responses coming from their inner wisdom. The more a person disconnects from him- or herself, the more that person becomes like an untuned car, driving down the freeway of life with black exhaust trailing behind.

Rather than being *selfish*, to cultivate pure *being* time is *selfull*. Thich Nhat Hanh, Buddhist monk, activist, and insightful author, once did a twist on the old phrase, "Don't just sit there, do something." He said, "Don't just do something, sit there!" He was inviting us into the truth that our value comes not from what we do or accomplish but from who we are. We can only know the depth of who we are when we spend time with ourselves. For many of us it means that we need to simplify our lives, for to live from the joy of being, we need to make spending time with ourselves a priority. I live in a beautiful 1914 cottage that looks out on a magical garden. Once a month, people come for a half day of silence. They climb the maple tree and feel it holding them. They sit by the waterfall, allowing its music to soothe them. They swing on the swing, watching the multitude of birds dance through the yard. By the time they leave, their eyes have regained their sparkle and their skin is glowing.

Taking time for ourselves is not only for us but also for everybody in our lives. How can we possibly live skillfully if we are not connected to ourselves? Rather than being self-indulgent, cultivating time where we can just *be* supports our loved ones and everyone else. Rather than being selfish, it is the greatest gift we can give to others — to listen to and live from our center. As we learn to nourish ourselves in this way, we can then give from a full tank, and our giving blesses everybody we touch. As we see through all the ideas that prevent us from being, it becomes clear not only that we have the right to *being* time but also that it is one of the core responsibilities of our lives. The more we become connected to ourselves, drinking from our inner wellspring, the less vulnerable we will be to a wave of compulsion. The less we are caught in compulsion's grip, the more we can know the joy that is our true nature. We then become life celebrating life, and everyone benefits from our "knowing and glowing."

The Joy of Being

Now that we know that it is safe and important to come home to ourselves, let us explore how to bring this wonderful healing experience into our lives. It is all about bringing our attention to our lives, not as we wish them to be, but exactly as they are, right here, right now. Remember the little girl in chapter 2 who kept being drawn back to the wonder of the river? She was *here*, connected with her life as it was in that moment. Because of that, she could feel the joy of the water in her whole being.

To know ourselves again with our birthright of aliveness and joy, we need to retrain ourselves to be fascinated with the experience of being alive. It is not about doing anything. It is just about being curious about what is happening right now. It is about being in our bodies; it is about being in our lives. It is relearning how to wash the dishes when we wash the dishes, to eat when we eat, and to hear when we are listening, so we can tap into the river of aliveness that is life. It is possible to be this alive in the middle of our busy lives.

Moments when we are fully here are powerfully healing. Jon Kabat-Zinn, in his book *Full Catastrophe Living*,[4] speaks about a study done at the University of Ohio. Exploring the effects of a high-fat, high-cholesterol diet on rabbits, researchers put these cuddly bundles of energy in cages stacked one on the other. When the test results came back, the rabbits in the lower cages had much less heart disease. This didn't make sense. They were all genetically identical, were on the same diet, and, it was thought, were being treated in the same way. That is, until it was discovered that the rabbits in the lower cages were periodically being taken out of the cages by one of the members of the team to be stroked, cuddled, and talked to.

A few moments of connection made a huge difference in the cholesterol level of the rabbits. This amazes us, but that is what *being* is all about. It is about connection. It is about choosing to be open to life, right here, right now — not an idea of it, but the real thing. And whether it is connection with a bunny hug, the beat of our heart, the taste of our food, the sound of a bird, the face of a loved one, or the warmth of the sun on our leg, this kind of connection heals.

Since we have been contained and controlled for so many years, how do we open to life again, cultivating the exhilaration of being? We laid the foundation by exploring a Returning Practice in chapter 7. Every time we bring our attention back to what is, we are cultivating being. Then in chapter 8 we learned to soften and open the contraction in our minds and bodies by touching whatever is there with the mercy of our hearts. In chapter 9 we explored how to open, ground, and connect through our breath.

The easiest way to weave all those things together is simply to pause for a few moments throughout your day, take a deep breath, briefly hold your breath, and then let go to your out-breath. You can even say silently to yourself (or out loud) the great sound of letting go: *ahhhh.* On this out-breath, let go of any pockets of chronic tension — the clenching in your jaw, the tightness in your shoulders, the contraction in your stomach, the tension in your feet. Imagine them melting like an ice cube placed in the sun. Really enjoy this letting go. Then, allow the next in-breath to open you from the inside out. The more you do this, the more you will be able to feel the tingles and aliveness in your body that are the field of joy. After you have grounded in your body, then open your attention to include everything around you. This is it! This is your life! Every moment of your journey has brought you to this moment, and this is the only one that matters. Receive it. See it. Hear it. Feel it. By being this present you are celebrating the gift of being alive!

I call moments like this the "pause that refreshes." In these pauses you are moving from unconsciousness to consciousness — from being caught in your head to being present with *what is right now.* At the beginning these pauses may not seem like much — just a few moments here and there. But I assure you they are much more powerful than all the zillions of moments you have been lost in your head. Stephen Levine once said that a life in which you experience even a few moments a day of fully being *here* is a life of healing.

Let me share an experience that demonstrates what I am talking about. Having just returned from a full weekend of teaching, I had a few hours the next morning to write. I found my mind fuzzy and my body very tired. I knew what I wanted to say, but it wouldn't come out in an orderly fashion. In the middle of my muddle, my cat jumped up on my lap, asking for my attention. Of course, my response was resistance. "I am doing some important work now," I said, "and I don't have time for you!"

As I continued to go round and round in my mind about what to write, my cat gently but persistently kneaded my legs, saying to me, "Take a break! Get out of your mind and come back into this moment." When I finally was able to see that I was a ball of resistance and could recognize the invitation my cat was giving me, I started to chuckle as I turned off the computer and curled up with her. Her purrs vibrated in my body, inviting me to soften my belly and come back into the delicious rhythm of my breath.

As I settled in, letting go of all the reactions in my mind, my attention filled my whole body, and there to meet me from the top of my head to the bottom of my toes was pure aliveness. The best word I can use to describe what I was experiencing was *delight*. When I was back in my body, the wisdom of the wellspring within filled me with its presence. As my kitty and I purred together (with a few kitty kisses here and there), the deep knowing that permeates this radiance revealed to me what wanted to be written with such clarity that I became amazed that I had stayed caught in my struggling mind for so long.

Moments such as these are powerful beyond your wildest imaginings. They are about nourishing yourself in the deepest way a human being can — with pure connection. The more you connect in this way, the less interesting your compulsion will be. In the middle of your day, you may not always be able to make full contact with life, but know that your aliveness is there, waiting for you. Just taking a few deep breaths, then bringing your attention back to yourself and then back to life will pave the way to a full and complete connection.

Practices for Cultivating the Joy of Being

What would it be like if you could learn to fill your body with delight rather than food, drugs, hectic busyness, or alcohol? What would it be like even in the middle of a busy day periodically to let go of your doing mind so you could tap into the connection and wisdom of simply *being?* As you understand the power of being and as you learn how to pay attention to life, you will see that it provides you with moments of downtime throughout your day. These are moments where you can cultivate pauses that refresh, connecting you with the healing of simply being. You may be waiting at the post office, frustrated with how long the line is, and suddenly you remember to connect. Close your eyes, take a few deep breaths, and let your tension melt as you feel your body. Listen to the symphony of sounds swelling and receding all around you, listening as if this is your first day on Earth. If you are in a bathtub, close your eyes, giving yourself to the water. Really melt. Then move your legs so the water swirls around you and open to the experience of its soothing embrace. When you are exercising, stop for a moment here and there and bring your full attention into your body. Really feel how exercise amplifies the river of aliveness. These pauses are moments of pure experience — immediate contact with life. You don't need to make a big production of this. Just a few breaths is often enough to get the ball rolling. For underneath all your wanting and fearing, trying and doing, is a longing to simply be present for this moment!

As you practice moments of being, your attention will become more finely tuned. No matter where you are, you will be able to feel the river of aliveness that fills your whole body right there underneath your chronic tightening and resistance to life. Becoming this connected to yourself you will then become much more of a human *being* rather than a human *doing.*

At the beginning as you pause you may recognize mostly your chronic tension and resistance to life. Don't fight it. To move out of reaction ask, "For this moment, can I let this be here?" This reminds you that fighting whatever is going on usually makes it worse. Then, for at least a couple of breaths, let it be and simply open to life. Just be willing to breathe through your tension and come back to being present for your surroundings. The joy will make itself known when it is ready.

Because softening and opening back into pure contact is so alien to most of us, it can be helpful to expand our capacity to *be* in more ways than just taking a few deep breaths here and there. We can set aside some time every day when we let go of all the outer demands and use our attention to connect. If your mind says you don't have enough time, that is just gobbledygook! Everything works better when we connect. If you truly feel that everything on your to-do list is absolutely essential, ask yourself if it will matter in a hundred years. It is amazing how that idea can cut through so much superfluous activity, bringing us back to the most essential thing — connection with life right here, right now.

I try every day to have "timeless time" in my garden. I swing on the swing, allowing my body to feel the joy of the rocking just as I did as a child. I will often close my eyes and just revel in these moments of pure connection. As I keep on swinging, I listen to the music of life — airplanes appearing and disappearing, birds calling to one another, the pleasant cacophony of passing cars, the thrill of the wind playing with the trees. There is no leaning into the future or wandering back into the past. There isn't any need for life (including me) to be any different from what it is.

In cultivating being time, choose something you enjoy. The word *enjoy* means "in joy!" Look for whatever brings more space into your mind and more lightness into your heart. What makes you feel warm and safe? What brings a smile to your face? What causes your belly to soften? (A soft belly is one of the clearest indicators that we are opening again to the river of aliveness that is life.) A wonderful question to ask is, "Right now, what do I *truly* need?" (We'll work more with this question in later chapters.) Is it curling up under the covers and melting into the experience? Is it renting a rowboat early on a Sunday morning and floating in the sounds and sights of awakening to another day? Is it asking your lover to give you a massage that won't lead to intercourse so you can practice melting into your body? Whatever it is, see if you are willing to give yourself at least a few minutes every day that are all about purely connecting with you and with life.

In the beginning, most of us return and open to *what is* only sporadically, and when we do, we become like bouncing balls — a moment of pure connection with life — then off we go back into the story in our heads. For a while, this is all we can do. We didn't learn how to walk overnight. We won't relearn how to come home to ourselves and life overnight either. But know that every time we return, we strengthen the muscle of our attention, increasing our capacity to be present. Then there comes a time when we are ready for more, ready to truly open to life again. It is when our whole body begins to remember that it is safe and healing to open that we can begin to live from *being*, tapping into its many treasures.

In opening to life you will be opening not only to the joy of being alive but also to the pains. You cannot have one without the other. When pain becomes something to embrace rather than resist, our moments of pain become healing. Every time you meet your pain in mercy, not only do you heal yourself, but you also lift the veil of forgetting that we all carry, making it easier for all beings to make the journey back to themselves. The following meditation will show you the power of meeting your pain.

Exercise

After you read through this exercise, close your eyes and take a few of those precious deep breaths that invite your whole body to let go. As you settle into the rhythm of your breath, allow yourself to become aware of one of the deeper pains of your life. It could be the sorrow of death, a cloud of depression, a feeling of being an outsider, the deep grief of being abandoned by a loved one, a debilitating physical challenge, a core feeling of shame.

Now expand your awareness and recognize that right now tens of thousands of people are experiencing exactly what you are. Take the feeling of abandonment, for example. Allow yourself to know that without a doubt, somewhere on the Earth, there are young children right now who are being abandoned on a city street, left to fend for themselves. Feel the overwhelming terror, confusion, and grief of these children. Allow yourself to recognize the truth that you are not alone in your pain, no matter what it is.

What can you do? You can come back to yourself. Feel this same pain inside you, but for these few moments, don't react. Become conscious of your pain. Become merciful with your pain. Meet it right here and right now. As you touch your pain through your merciful attention, you can finally recognize that this is not just your pain. It is the pain of humanity, and as you heal your pain with your merciful attention, you take the collective mind of humanity another step into healing. Now find others on the Earth who are experiencing the same pain. There are many. You are not alone. Feel their pain inside of you and know that you can truly make a difference by being present for yourself, exactly as you are.

At first glance, this may not appear to make much of a difference. Instead, you may want to go buy an airplane ticket and go help all those people in pain. But when you meet the pain within you — the pain that we all carry, the pain that causes each one of us to live in unskillful ways — you literally help to heal the pain of the world. This may seem like only a drop in a mighty ocean of pain, but drop-by-drop it can be healed.

This meditation also works with our joy. Because you are a part of the web of life, every time you are present, tasting your food, seeing your lover's face, feeling the cool evening air on your cheek, you bring the collective mind of humanity another step into conscious and loving connection with life. It is empowering, not only for you but also for every person on Earth, for you to take time to be with yourself exactly as you are. May all beings be free from suffering. May all beings know peace.

Some Helpful Hints

In the past when we have tried to cultivate *being,* oftentimes we have experienced it just in our heads. How many times have you had a massage during which you were up in your head wishing that the therapist would do things a little differently? Or what about during sex — are you really present, or are you reviewing the shopping list in your head? And how many times have you floated in a warm bath, with candles, no less, and read a book? I am not saying that is bad. All I am saying is that who you are is not a thought, it is an experience!

When you understand that, then you will be ready to take another step — a step into truly experiencing what you are experiencing. Remember that the intellect will try to take over. Before opening to being, it may say, "I am afraid to be with me." "I can't hear what I need." "I don't have time." "I had an awful day." "I don't know how to do this." "I won't do it right." "I am too depressed." "I am too empty." "I am too sick." "I am too out of touch." "I am too tired." "I am too unworthy, fat, or ugly." "I have too many people depending on me to take care of me." (And the big one) "I do not deserve to feel joy in my life."

You will always be running up against the next reason why you can't or won't open to being. *All your resistances are actually very good reasons to be present for yourself.* This is when you most need yourself. When we are pressed to the max by our lives, disconnected from ourselves, we all feel vulnerable, whether or not we can acknowledge it. Just as an overwhelmed or overly tired child needs to be taken care of, so does our vulnerability. It is soothed and supported when we come back to ourselves. If we are stretched to the limit, we need to return to ourselves in simple and nourishing ways.

The intellect also may be so enamored of the joy of being that instead of being present, it is planning how you can do more of this in your life. Or it may get sidetracked into judging how well you are doing. It may even tell you this is boring and isn't doing anything for you. Rather than listening to your thoughts, use them as an indicator that you have again left contact with *your immediate experience.* Pause. Take a few deep breaths and come back to curiosity about what you are experiencing right now.

As we cultivate the river of joy and aliveness that is life, the final thing we need to remember is that we may be afraid of being. We have been contained and controlled for so long that we have forgotten the safety, the nourishment, and the exhilaration of opening to life. Not only are we unfamiliar with it, but we don't know what to do with it. The mind often turns on the *control mode* when aliveness floods us with its truth. "Hold on for a minute. Where is the shut-off valve? I need to be in control here."

So we need to explore opening to life in little bites, slowly expanding our capacity for the joy of being alive. It is also important to recognize that our capacity for free-flowing joy is like a clogged-up old pipe. When we start allowing the water through it again, it will happen in fits and starts as it pushes out all the contraction in our bodies, minds, and hearts. Remember that as you are clearing out your "pipes," you are heading for the clear-flowing water of your own vitality.

A Few More Practices

Give yourself permission at least to contemplate your right to the joy of being. In this contemplation, if you don't see clearly how you could cultivate being, I offer a few other ways to get the juices flowing. Each of them is about spending time away from outer demands so that you can cultivate a deep and nourishing relationship with yourself and with life. I am not giving them to you as another thing to add to your already full to-do list. I offer these ideas more as triggers to get your imagination going. Listen carefully to your body as you read them, and it will show which ones it wants to explore.

• Give yourself a face massage. Every inch of your skin contains nineteen thousand sensory cells! Soothe your brow, cradle your cheek, tap your forehead, ruffle your eyebrows, explore your lips. Or ask a friend for a foot massage.

- Whenever you find yourself waiting in line, bring your attention back into your body, take a few deep breaths, and open to the preciousness of this moment.

- Turn off all the lights and bathe or shower in the dark.

- Lie on the grass and allow yourself to be held by the Earth. Make sand castles at the beach. Buy an air mattress and float on the water. Climb a tree.

- Rather than a sick day, take a "well day" from work. Pretend that you are your best friend who wants to give you a day full of delight, whether it is a day in nature or a day in bed.

- Have an "I don't have to do it day." Don't exercise, don't floss your teeth, don't return phone calls. Disconnect from the enslavement of *doing*.

- Move your body without thinking of it as exercise. Do log rolls down a hill, swing on a swing, go dancing, run for the pure joy of it, jump on a trampoline. Our bodies love to move!

- Go to a public place with sights and smells that bring you joy. It could be a playground with the happy sounds of children, a coffee shop filled with warm smells and the delightful murmur of people connecting with one another, a library with the wonderful smell of books and the fullness of silence. Imagine that tomorrow you will suddenly become blind and deaf. Allow this idea to open you to really savoring this experience for the preciousness that it truly is. Nothing is ordinary.

- If certain feelings are blocking your access to simply *being*, exaggerate them. If you are mad, stomp around and get wild. If you are feeling sorry for yourself, turn up the whine dial and ham it up. If you are afraid, comfort yourself as if you were your only child. If you are grieving, rent a sad movie, get a box of Kleenex, and have a good cry. Don't minimize even the smallest of griefs. And if you're just stuck, go howl at the moon or sing loudly in your car.

- Make a comfort nest somewhere in your home. Nourish your body with soft, cushy, warm stuff. Then breathe yourself back into openness, using one of the breath techniques we have explored.

- If you want to overeat, listen to yourself, discover what food you are craving, and place it in front of you. If it isn't clear exactly what you want, choose any food. Smell it, explore it with your eyes, and discover it with your touch. When you are ready, allow yourself to take one bite and play with it like you did when you were a child. Roll it around in your mouth and explore it with your tongue. (Tongues love to play!) When you are ready, bite into it and allow its essence to flow across your taste buds. Become enamored of the pleasures of taste. Be stunned by how satisfying one bite of food can be. People often speak about how satiated they are by a small amount of food when they are present for the experience.

- Nourish your sight with beauty — a picture or a tiny vase of flowers. Discover what would nourish your ears — wind chimes or maybe a tape of ocean waves. Remind yourself that whenever you see or hear a gift of beauty, you will pause and reconnect with life, right here, right now.

- Don't speak for a whole day. Silence can be very nourishing, grounding, and connecting.

- Slowly, with great tenderness, bring your hand over your heart and touch yourself with mercy.

Don't ever forget that you have permission to feel this good and are worthy of this kind of time and attention. As you learn how to return to yourself, feeding yourself from the inside out and filling yourself with the joy of being, the temporary pleasure of compulsion that so quickly turns into devastation will take a back seat. You will finally be free. Enjoy the ride!

Now that we have explored the four skills of engagement, let us bring them together by learning how to use four questions in our hunt for all the treasures hidden inside our compulsions.

Core Ideas

- When we feel disconnected from ourselves and our lives, compulsions become a substitute for the true joy of coming home to ourselves.

- *Being* is composed of moments when your mind, body, and heart are all in the same place at the same time.

- Not only is it safe to open to life, but it is only in opening to whatever is right here, right now that we will discover the connection and the peace that we long for.

- If we open to our pain in curiosity, we bring it out of the shadows into the light where we can work with it in kind and skillful ways.

- Our bodies are a gift from life. They are nothing less than magnificent, no matter what shape, size, color, or age.

- As you learn how to feed yourself from the inside out, filling yourself with the joy of *being,* the temporary pleasure of compulsions will take a backseat and you will know the healing that you long for.

- The greatest gift we can give to others is to take time to simply be, to listen to and live from our center. As we learn to nourish ourselves in this way, we can then give from a full tank, and our giving blesses everybody we touch.

- When you were young, you were naturally in contact with how delicious it was to have a body. You lived inside your body, inside yourself, and you were in touch daily with your inner well-spring.

- Every time you are present for whatever is going on in your body, you are taking another step into living *in* your body, connected to the river of aliveness that is you.

- It is possible to be this alive in the middle of our busy lives. It is not about doing anything. It is just about being curious about life as it is right now. It is about being in our bodies; it is about being in our lives.

- Our bodies are constantly speaking to us, giving us the clues to our healing. As you return to your body, you will know your rightful heritage of joy and aliveness.

PART FOUR

TREASURE
Hunting

Chapter 11

PREPARING TO FIND THE

Treasure

The skills we explored in part 3 are about clearing a pathway from the maze of our minds back into an immediate, creative, trust-filled, and joyful connection with ourselves and our lives. As you incorporate these skills into your daily life, you may experience moments of pure connection with the field of *being* that you truly are. You may finally recognize that this is what you have been truly longing for, especially when you are compulsive. But you have probably discovered, on this journey back to yourself, thoughts and feelings within you that you dislike and even fear. And these old patterns — of fear, anger, confusion, self-judgment, sadness, loneliness — can be pretty seductive, taking over in a flash and throwing us back into the old world of reaction and struggle, which fuels our compulsions.

In this part of the book we will bring everything we have explored together into four questions that we can use to transform all these old patterns and the challenges they bring into our lives — especially our compulsions. These questions will deepen your experience of everything we have explored so far in the book. They will allow you to see what is fueling your compulsion and then to transform it through the light of your compassionate attention. And finally, they will help you tap into what you are truly longing for whenever you are compulsive.

This powerful way of transforming (rather than always trying to fix) our compulsions is new for most of us. And we all feel a little trepidation in turning toward ourselves rather than endlessly turning away. Even Oprah Winfrey experienced this fear. While talking with Gary Zukav, author of *The Seat of the Soul*,[1] she clearly revealed our strong belief that if we just stayed in control we would know the peace we long for. The show that day was on addictions, and she was speaking about the night that she ate lots of macaroni and cheese and bread pudding after seeing the negative reviews of her movie *Beloved*. While sharing with Gary, she began to see that she didn't just want to eat that night. She was also trying to run away from feelings of powerlessness and rejection.

Gary helped her to see why it is so important to meet our feelings. When she was invited to go deeper, Oprah immediately talked about management techniques, saying that she could have gone for a run or to the gym. Gary invited her to *feel* what was going on inside her. In other words, he invited her to engage with her experience rather than trying to manage it. She expressed the resistance we all feel to doing this by saying how much just remembering that night brought up painful feelings for her. She then said, "Why would I want to sit there and feel all of that?" Gary responded, "Because if you don't, you will need to contend with this very strong impulse to eat, gamble, buy, run, drink, have sex."

To start responding to our experience rather than always living in reaction, we need to be reminded over and over again to bring the light of our compassionate attention to what we are experiencing. For two very important reasons, I call this ability to be present for our immediate experience "treasure hunting." The first reason is that *treasures are always hidden in the sensations, feelings, and thoughts that we have habitually run from.*

If we look closely we will notice life's inclination to hide its treasures in the dark. We have alluded to this truth in the stories we pass down through the generations. In practically every one of our myths, both the keys to the adventure and the treasures themselves are usually hidden in the dark: the dragon sits on the golden egg. The princess is protected by a moat full of crocodiles. The evil queen possesses the magic wand. The necessity of the dark — of the difficult, challenging aspects of our lives — is woven through Homer's *Odyssey,* Dante's *Inferno,* and even *The Wizard of Oz.* Each of the main characters in that movie became more of themselves through their challenges — the lion discovered his courage, the scarecrow his intelligence, the tin man his heart, and Dorothy her way home.

Our compulsions and the boxed-up feelings that fuel them are where the treasures of our true self are hidden. *To discover what lies hidden under our compulsions, we need to learn how to turn toward our experience rather than away.* "No. No. Never!" we say. As Oprah asked, "Why would I ever want to do that?" Suspend your resistance for a moment and imagine a huge and ferocious lion chasing you. This is what it is like with the boxed-up feelings within us that we have tried to escape through our compulsions. When the lions of these feelings come close to the surface, we put on our running shoes and sprint. We eat more chocolate, find more things to do, surf the Internet, get out our credit cards.

Sometimes you can outdistance the lion. Eventually, if you are lucky, you won't be able to run anymore. Falling to the ground, you are sure you are going to be devoured. As the lion screeches to a halt beside you, much to your amazement, he doesn't even take a bite out of you. Instead, he turns into a pussycat, and as his mouth opens, you see resting on his tongue a gift he has been trying to deliver for years! The lion is your compulsion and all the feelings you have been running from. And just like the lion, these feelings hold great treasures. But you have to stop running to be gifted by them.

The second reason I call this process treasure hunting is that as we meet ourselves with curiosity and compassion instead of turning away, all the boxed-up parts of ourselves can be transformed back into the free-flowing aliveness they came from. Remember in chapter 4, when I invited you to shake your body, all the tingles and aliveness you felt everywhere? That was a tiny glimpse into the kind of joy that is our birthright. Instead of being fully alive, we are like water that has turned into ice. As we bring the light of our attention into what we are experiencing, the ice of our struggles begins to thaw into flowing water. Then, as we give ourselves the warm light of our heart, our struggles evaporate into the air just like water evaporating into steam. We then become one again with the field of being that is life. This kind of transformation comes when we realize that what we are experiencing isn't as important as our *relationship* to what we are experiencing.

In chapter 12, "The Healing Power of Questions," you will learn the power of asking questions and discover what kinds of questions will allow you to engage with and transform your immediate experience. In chapter 13, "Treasure Hunting with Sensations," you will be shown how to use these core tools to meet the sensations in your body, which initially is the easiest place to learn how to meet and transform your experience. In chapter 14, "Treasure Hunting with Feelings," you will discover how to use these techniques to meet the thoughts and feelings that have caused you to run to your compulsion(s) over and over. And finally, in chapter 15, "Treasure Hunting with Compulsions," you will learn how to bring everything we have explored so far to your compulsions so that you can heal them and be healed by them in the process.

We have now arrived at the most technical part of the book. Initially I invite you to read each chapter in this section, just to get a feeling for what is being offered. Then read each chapter again, watching for the techniques that feel most appropriate to you. Remember, you are the only person who knows what steps you need to take toward your healing.

Core Ideas

- Hidden in the inner experiences you habitually run from always lies a treasure.

- "Treasure hunting" is the ability to be compassionately present for our immediate experience. It is about bringing your attention to your life, not as you wish it to be, but exactly as it is, right here, right now.

- To discover the treasure that lies hidden under our compulsions, we need to learn how to turn toward our experience.

- As we meet ourselves with curiosity and compassion instead of turning away, all our boxed-up feelings can be transformed back into the free-flowing aliveness they came from.

- Transformation comes when we realize that what we are experiencing isn't as important as our *relationship to* what we are experiencing.

Chapter 12

THE HEALING POWER OF

Questions

L iving in questions is one of the most powerfully transformative tools available to us, and we are only beginning to tap into its power. No matter where we are, no matter what is happening, living in questions can bring clarity when we are confused, courage when our strength has failed us, hope when we are filled with despair, and vision when we don't have a clue about which way to go. These questions can also transform not only the sensations and feelings that are fueling our compulsions but also our compulsions themselves.

Notice that I use the words *living in questions*. That is different from just *asking* questions. Our old way — ask a question and look for the answer — is necessary in our day-to-day lives. But asking questions in this way can often bring us frustration, especially when we ask them about our compulsions. That was certainly my experience. Looking for answers about why I was compulsive and how I could stop was exhausting, confusing, and frustrating. Most of the time I couldn't find the answers I was looking for. If I did, I usually couldn't hold on to them, or they became obsolete. It was when I learned how to ask questions in a different way that the clouds began to lift and I was able to start healing.

This chapter is about a new way of working with questions in which we discover that the power of questions is not in finding the answers that we are looking for. Rather, *the power of questions lies in the questions themselves.* There are two ways to tap into this power. The first way is using what I call "check-in" questions. This type of question is about bringing our attention into our immediate experience so that we can calm down our reactive mind. In this calming, we can see what is really going on and create enough space within us so that we can listen to the wellspring of deeper knowing that is always present. The second way of tapping into the power of questions is using what I call "open-ended" questions. This type of question is about asking questions without looking for a specific answer. Through this powerful way of working with questions, answers come to us from beyond our own limited understanding. We can use each type of question to treasure hunt with our compulsions and the sensations and feelings that are fueling them.

Although treasure hunting with questions is a very fluid and alive process, for clarity and simplicity we will work with four basic questions that encompass the skills we explored earlier. We will first look at them as check-in questions, which allow us to meet and transform whatever experiencing we are having. We will then explore how to transform each question into its open-ended version so that we can ask to receive help and clarity about whatever is going on in our life.

We will also note the intent of each of the questions so that you can better understand how to use them in your healing. I have worked with these four questions with many people over the years, and, based on this experience, I have worded them carefully to bring forth the core intention of each of them. When you are clear about their intent and have become familiar with working with questions, you will discover your own questions. You can also draw from the list of other questions at the end of this chapter, listening for the ones that call to you. Let us now explore the four check-in questions.

Check-in Questions

Check-in questions take us out of the reactive mind, inviting us into the healing of response. They focus our attention on our immediate experience in a spacious and curious way, tapping us into the wellspring of our own deep knowing. The first check-in question invites us into the power of curiosity, the second the openness of spaciousness, the third the healing of compassion, and the fourth the power of listening to our own wisdom. Each of these questions allows us literally to transform our compulsions and the sensations and feelings fueling them so that we can again know the field of joy that we are.

In This Moment, What Am I Experiencing?

As we have explored throughout this book, the healing we long for begins when we can be curious about what is happening right now. That is why the first question is so powerful. It dips the finger of our attention into the river of our experience. Rather than leaving us lost in reaction, it invites us to be curious about what is happening right now so we can see the truth of what we are experiencing. This is the primary question, for it is both the means and the end to our healing. It brings us into deep connection with ourselves and our lives, which is, after all, what we most want. It also helps us to see and dissolve anything that stands in the way of this pure connection.

Most of us have a tendency to look at what we don't like about our lives and then to get lost in how we can make it better. In other words, we are geared to making things into problems, and we have the capacity to struggle with practically everything. We want what we don't have, and we usually don't want what we do have. Constantly wanting things to be different, we don't see that our lives, rather than being a random series of events, are living adventures, offering us the exact experiences we need to grow into the fullness of our potential.

The intent of this question is to help us cultivate curiosity, and it is this curiosity that cuts through our wanting things to be different than what they are. It allows us to let go of the story about what we are experiencing so that we can actually experience it. Then we can passionately listen to our lives. In this listening, we discover that every experience contains valuable information that can help us immensely in our healing. When we are willing to look at and then experience what is going on, everything that happens adds to our healing rather than feeding our old urge to struggle. The tight knot in the stomach, the lump in the throat, the anger that feels like it is going to explode are all trying to tell us something. They are messengers from the deepest and wisest parts of ourselves, and they come bearing information and insights that will help us dissolve the reactions that fuel our compulsions.

In the next three chapters we will explore how to take this question into our inner experience, where we can use it to see and let go of all the thoughts and feelings that fuel our compulsions. For now, work with it as you did in chapter 7, by becoming fascinated by what is happening in your life right now. As you ask, "In this moment, what am I experiencing?" you can focus on the sounds all around you, the play of shadow and light, the face of whomever you are talking to, the wide range of colors and shapes, or the taste of your food. When your attention drifts back into your head, to your story about life, say to yourself, "ahh, thinking, thinking" and let the story go so you can bring your attention back to the immediacy of life. The more you cultivate present-moment awareness, the more you will see that there is a big difference between being identified with your story *about* life and being present for life *as it is.* This process begins to awaken within you not only the longing to be present for life but also the desire to see and dissolve all the old stories within you that keep you cut off from the joy of being fully alive.

This is when you can begin to use this question to become familiar with all the old patterns within you that keep you separate. When an old story of fear, sadness, or anger arrives, simply ask this question, acknowledge what is going on within you, and then *let it go.* Your life then becomes a fluid dance in which you have no need either to hold on to or to resist whatever you are experiencing.

In the beginning of our awakening, all of us have so much within that we haven't met and healed through the light of our compassionate attention. So when we bring our attention to our immediate experience, instead of being able to see and let go of what is going on inside us, we may experience confusion, frustration, and resistance. The next three questions are what I call processing questions. You can use them when you can't open back into life because your reactive patterns are stronger than your ability to see them and let them go. These questions can help immensely in meeting and then dissolving old patterns so you can be fully connected to life again.

For This Moment, Can I Let This Be Here?

The first question is all about recognizing what we are experiencing right now and then letting go of anything that stands in the way of a full connection with life. Sometimes we experience turbulence in our minds and hearts that we can't open to or let go of. This is the time to open to the intention of this second question — to allow whatever is there to be there. As we've seen over and over, *the quickest and most powerful way to dissolve our struggles is to let them be.* By now we are starting to understand that resisting something we are experiencing only gives it more energy. If we can accept our experience, and then be willing to look and listen, whatever we are experiencing loses its power over us. Letting something be also understands that most everything we experience is temporary. Everything in life arises and passes away. Even though our most painful experiences come with the thought that they will be here forever, it is never true. They fade too, just as night always fades into day. Letting somthing be allows whatever is there to flow through us rather than staying static.

The healing power of letting something *be* is built on the truth that when we tighten around life and resist, we hurt more; when we soften and open, we hurt less. Our controlling minds resist this new way of being with ourselves only until they see the magic that can happen when we let things be. The Beatles alluded to this magic in their song *Let It Be.*

There are two important points to grasp in understanding the phenomenal power of letting something be. First, letting something be isn't about being a helpless victim. Rather, it helps us to reclaim our power.

It does this by taking us out of reactive mode so we can look and explore, becoming fascinated with what is going on. To access the power of this second question we need to understand that our lives are not a random series of events meant to confound, upset, or even please us. Each experience we have is tailor-made to show us the doorway back into the joy of pure *being*. Second, letting something be is not about not *doing* anything. We often do what is called a "duality flip" when we hear about letting something be. Since letting something be isn't about controlling, we think it must mean the opposite — that you just sit on the side of the road of life and let it all happen to you. Nothing could be further from the truth. Letting something be is about letting go of the reactive mode so that we can respond instead. And response is a very creative place to live from.

A great example of the clarity and empowerment this second question can bring came from a woman in one of my groups who began working with this question in her challenging relationship. Her partner was a very controlling man, and this would bring up deep rage inside her. Because he wasn't yet a safe person with whom she could speak her rage, she found herself constantly on "pre-boil." This subterranean anger was beginning to show up as physical difficulties in her body.

When she began asking the questions, she was amazed at the depth of her anger. The first question allowed her to take her attention off her partner and bring it back to herself. As she let go of her *story about* what was going on, she could become curious about what was happening inside her. At first the idea of letting the anger *be* was alien to her, because she had been taught to fight it her whole life. But with a little coaxing, asking the second question created enough space inside her that she could begin to listen to her anger. The next time we talked, her eyes were sparkling as she said, "I have never listened to my anger before. I could truly experience it without getting lost in it! As I acknowledged it and listened to what it had to say, I watched it fade away. I was then much clearer about what I needed to say and do in the relationship that would be healing for both of us."

This story shows us that cultivating the ability to let things be isn't about being powerless. It is about moving out of reaction so that we can respond clearly and cleanly to life. And responding isn't about being a wimp. Rather, our response can have a clear, sharp edge that cuts through muddle like a samurai's sword. This story also reminds us that letting go cannot transform anything that you haven't accepted as a part of you. Remember, in the story about the house of your being from chapter 2, all the parts of us that were boxed up and hidden away? Over and over they got out of their boxes, padded up the stairs to the attic, and knocked on the door of our mind. Over and over again we rejected, ignored, or shamed them. When we learn to open the door and let them into our awareness (the first question) and then accept them as a part of us (the second question), then and only then can the light of our compassionate attention transform them. Remember, this is a process of "meeting" our feelings rather than just feeling them. The foundation for this meeting is what this second question is all about.

When you begin to bring this question into the challenges of your life, you may find yourself answering it with a no: "No. I don't want this headache or this anxiety or my craving to be here." But this is workable too. That is the beauty of the questions. If you answer no, simply go back to the first question and ask, "In this moment, what am I experiencing?" What you will recognize is that you are resisting being present for what you are experiencing. You can then ask the second question again, for if you can let go of struggling with your resistance to being with your experience, whatever you are experiencing loses its power over you. Simply go back and forth between the two questions until you can find something you can allow to be. When your answer is yes, the clouds of reaction will lift.

At times you won't be able to find a yes. That's okay. If you find that you are completely resisting your experience, you can ask a variation of the second question: "For this moment, can I not struggle with this?" Remember, whatever you resist persists. To accept that this is what you are experiencing lets you reclaim your power. Know that the inclusiveness of this question works like magic. It can transform the hardest heart, the deepest grief, and the sharpest pain. Under its influence, our bodies soften, our hearts let go, and our attention becomes a healing force for our highest good.

In This Moment, Can I Touch This with Compassion?

At the center of all great spiritual teachings lies the knowledge that everything is truly healed in the heart. Respected writers, great spiritual leaders, inspired poets, and children all remind us that mercy, kindness, understanding, compassion, and love are what life is all about. The reason heart energy is so powerful is that it doesn't hate or fear what it focuses on. Instead, it brings understanding to whatever you are experiencing, and in this spaciousness and inclusion, things are transformed.

I wrote a powerful story in my first book that speaks of a time when, in the midst of a great challenge, I was able to meet myself in my own heart. I signed up for a retreat called "African Drumming, Dancing, Ritual and Art." On the first evening, I began to get an inkling of what I was in for. There was no schedule, and I never had any idea when meals would be served. A transformer had blown just before we arrived, so there was no hot water, heat, or lights in the cabins and very little warmth in the big, drafty hall. At three in the morning on the second night, after having gone through many phases of a ritual, the leaders left without any indication of when they would return.

Up to this point, I had checked in with myself repeatedly and had decided that it was important to stay with the retreat. But now, in the middle of the night, exhausted and cold, sitting on a hard floor with no end in sight, I wanted to leave. Panic began to build in my body and mind as I was pushed to my limit and I felt like I was going to explode. Awareness was obscured by a mixture of terror, despair, and self-hatred. "I can't handle this. When is it going to be over? I should have left. I am so inept. And besides, I'm such a wimp," my old voices screamed at me. Then curiosity kicked in. I asked a variation of the first question, "What *is?*" and my attention came out of reaction and back into the living experience, recognizing overwhelm, exhaustion, and fear. Calming myself through responding to my immediate experience, I remembered that my life is a journey of awakening in which everything is grist for the mill of becoming conscious. I then asked an open-ended version (which we'll get to in a bit) of the first question, "What is asking to be met?"

Under the light of my compassionate attention, memories of other times in my life when I had felt caught in an overwhelming situation with no way out and no end in sight came flooding into my awareness. But for the first time in my life, someone was there meeting me in this indescribably painful place. And that someone was *me*.

I began to talk to this core feeling of "no way out." As I asked the third question, "In this moment, can I touch this with compassion?" my heart opened. I could say to the terror, "It's okay. I understand." Rather than becoming caught in reaction, my heart cradled these feelings with a deep sense of tenderness and mercy. This softening and inclusion warmed my body. When sensations of cold or panic began to seep back in, I found myself repeatedly returning to the warm glow of compassionate curiosity. As the room became colder, my heart became warmer. What had been an indescribably painful situation was transformed into one of the major healing experiences of my life. I knew as I packed to leave later that morning that I had been deeply opened and now trusted myself completely. I saw that even when I am pushed to the limit I am capable of being there for myself, touching my most painful parts of me with my heart.

My ability to be that present for myself on that cold floor in the wee hours of the morning came from the understanding that there is nothing inside me, or anybody else, that does not deserve compassion and understanding. And when our hearts finally open to ourselves, all that we have held in judgment and in fear can be transformed.

Right Now, What Do I Truly Need?

The intent of the fourth question is to help us listen. It not only invites us into a deeper level of listening to our experience, but it also awakens our wellspring of deep knowing. This is not a listening with our heads, but an internal listening to the wisdom within that knows what needs to happen to bring balance back into our lives.

To open to the intent of this question is much like being in a room with very loud music filling up the entire space and then suddenly hearing the music stop. There to greet you is the song of the bird outside the window, the hum of the refrigerator, the beat of your heart. All those were happening when the music was playing, but you couldn't hear them. The same is true of our own deep knowing. It is always speaking to us, but we can't hear it because of the static created by our reactions. Asking, "Right now, what do I *truly* need?" signals our willingness to listen.

A very important distinction needs to be made here. We are not asking for what we *want*. Wants come from the desire for immediate gratification, based on a limited perspective. Needs come from a deeper place that is in alignment with what is for our highest good. That is why the word *truly* is in italics. It invites us to listen to the deep wisdom within us. The dictionary defines *truly* as "accurately, genuinely, sincerely, rightfully." All these words allude to what we are talking about here. The dictionary also tells us that *true* comes from an ancient word meaning "basic sense" or "firm as a tree."

The most important thing about this question is the willingness to ask it. It is a doorway into discovering the kindest and most skillful thing we can do in any moment. Because most of us have not been taught how to truly listen to ourselves, at first nothing may come clear. If it doesn't, don't try to figure it out. That will just take you back up into your head. Know that turning toward yourself and asking this question is powerful in its own right. Also, asking the question awakens your inner wellspring, making it easier over time to hear exactly what will bring peace into your life.

Because we are not trained to listen to ourselves, it can be very helpful to work with this question when our lives are somewhat calm. Make a game of it. If you are sitting on the couch after dinner, check in with yourself and then ask, "Right now, what do I *truly* need?" Or maybe it is a hectic day at work and the candy machine is looking somewhat interesting. Instead of grabbing your purse, pause, check in with yourself, and then listen for the answer to the question, What do I *truly* need? Don't pressure yourself. You may simply need to get out of the building and walk around the block. Or you may not be able to hear your own wisdom at first. In the beginning, when all is not clear, know that just asking this question sets the answer in motion.

As we have seen, the four questions happen in a progression. The first brings curiosity into our immediate experience, the second opens a space around it, the third awakens our heart, and the fourth connects us to the wellspring of wisdom within us. But you don't have to use them in that order. Each question stands on its own, or you can combine them in any way that works for you.

Remember, the first question is the primary one, bringing us back into the living moment and highlighting everything that stands in the way of being present. If we can't let go of whatever is keeping us from being present, we can move on to any of the next three questions, understanding that they are specifically meant for transforming our experience through spaciousness, mercy, and wisdom. Listen to yourself. Get creative, and let the questions work their magic for you.

Open-Ended Questions

The second way of working with questions that can heal us to our core is to ask open-ended questions. In this type of question we are not looking for answers. Instead we are opening ourselves so that answers can come to us from the deepest and wisest parts of ourselves. Maybe you are saying, "You must be crazy. Ask a question and not look for an answer? That is insanity. I don't have time for this. I am too busy trying to figure it all out." But if you watch carefully, you will see that a quest for answers keeps you caught in your head, left only with your own limited understanding. Lost in the search for the answers to our lives, we have totally missed the power of the questions themselves.

The power of open-ended questions comes to us when we realize that life is a field of Intelligence. Everywhere we look, we see its handiwork, whether it is the dance of an electron, the play of the wind, or the laughter of a child. This Intelligence is beyond our limited human minds' ability to comprehend. If you doubt that, check in with your body. It is made up of more than one hundred trillion cells, and they all work together with barely a thought from you. Even to begin to grasp this astounding cooperation and creativity, imagine every person on Earth working with everybody else for the common good of the whole. Hard to imagine? But that wouldn't even begin to come close to what your body does. It would take over sixteen thousand Earths, each with 6 billion people, all working together, even to come close to what your body does every day.

Although we may not be able to comprehend the working of the vast Intelligence at the heart of life, we can partner with it through asking open-ended questions. We need to understand that though we don't *look* for the answer, we can still *expect* an answer. In fact, asking open-ended questions guarantees an answer. But if we look for the answer, we gum up the works. Let me explain.

When we ask a question without looking for an answer, it creates a vacuum that has to be filled. It is much like the process of canning peas. We put the peas in a jar, screw on the lid, and then place them in the boiling water to create the vacuum that seals the jar. Asking a question and then continually looking for the answer — "Is this it? No, but maybe this is it, I don't know the answer, this is too confusing" — is like lifting the jar out of the boiling water and taking off the lid to see if the vacuum has been created. Of course, now we have broken the seal and lost the vacuum. To ask a question and not look for the answer literally creates a vacuum in the universe. It is a law of physics. The Intelligence of the Universe rushes into the vacuum of an open-ended question, and the answer automatically, in its own time, condenses out of the void and into our lives.

Rather than asking open-ended questions of the vast Intelligence of life, we usually narrow ourselves down to our own limited resources and understanding. Give us the simplest of challenges in our lives, and rather than going into the spaciousness of an open-ended question, we go into struggle and a sense that we have to do it ourselves. We are like students sitting in a classroom doing a difficult math problem while an extraordinary teacher stands in front of the room. Instead of recognizing the teacher and asking skillful questions, we sit doubled over our books, struggling with the problem. Without even looking up, we desperately search for the answer, exhausting all the information we have and grappling with ever-increasing frustration. We can even slip into self-judgment and despair: "I'll never get through this." "I'm always stuck." "Everybody else gets it and I don't." Just think of your endless struggle with your compulsion, and you will see the truth of this analogy. Rather than engaging with our own deep knowing, we struggle with the struggle, never asking the "teacher within us" for help.

When I began to live in open-ended questions, a wonderful truth became clear to me: problems and solutions are two sides of the same coin, and they always show up together. The resolution to every problem we have ever had or ever will have is nestled in the heart of the challenge. Life waits for the spaciousness of a question. Asking this type of question signals the Universe that we are willing to listen to the truth and the wisdom that comes with every challenge in our lives. This type of question doesn't work in linear time — ask a question and get an answer. Answers will come in their own time and their own way. I've received them while reading a spy novel in which one sentence stands out from the rest, almost as if I were reading the whole book just to receive those few words. I've also overheard conversations in the grocery store in which a few words pierced my unknowing and answered my question. Answers come in dreams and even while I'm taking a shower or cooking dinner. They can come with startling clarity or arrive gradually like the dawning of a day.

Until I learned the power of open-ended questions, I was like a fish out of water. In so many situations, I didn't know what to do. I was raising two children by myself and, as I once told my oldest child, "I have never done this before!" I was also being stretched in my work in ways that sometimes scared me silly. The more I asked open-ended questions, the more I discovered a true partnership with a power that was a lot smarter than I. The clarity these questions bring was most evident in difficult situations. Whether it was a teenage daughter who decided she wasn't going to listen to anything I said or a client who was on the verge of suicide, when I asked for help through these questions, I was taken out of my panicked mind that was certain it didn't know the right thing to do or say and was then connected to a wisdom that was always and unfailingly clear. Once I created a partnership with these questions, I wondered how I ever survived without them.

I then began to ask open-ended questions about my compulsions. It astounds me now that it took me so long before I could bring these questions to my compulsions. Reflecting on this, I realized that my lack of faith that anything could heal my compulsion was so great that it probably would have chewed my questions up and spit them out in a flash. But by the time I started using questions when I was compulsive, I had had enough direct proof of their power that I knew they were working their magic even when it didn't seem like the questions were making a dent in the process.

The art of trusting that the Intelligence of the Universe will answer our questions comes to each of us in its own time and in its own way. Slowly we move beyond our doubt that the Universe awaits our questions. We then see through the subtle but very strong illusion that we are in charge, and finally we discover the patience to wait for the answers to come.

One of the wonderful things about using open-ended questions is that you don't have to know what is going on, what you are feeling, or even what kind of answer you want. You also don't have to have a concept of this Intelligence that is waiting for the opening of a question. You don't even have to trust that it will answer you. All you need to do is ask and let the question go, and the answer will show up in the vacuum created by your question. The beauty of asking open-ended questions, allowing the Universe to answer rather than relying on our own limited intelligence, is that we don't just *get* an answer. We *become* the answer itself. There is a huge difference between understanding something with our heads and understanding it with our whole *being*. The answer *lives* us. We then know a true partnership with life.

Now that we understand the power of open-ended questions, let us explore how to use them to tap into the nourishment, clarity, support, and love that we need on our journey back to ourselves. What we will be doing here is slightly changing each of the check-in questions, transforming them into their open-ended versions.

What Is Asking to Be Seen?

We transform our first check-in question, "In this moment, what am I experiencing?" into an open-ended question by asking, "What is asking to be seen?" This question is helpful to ask when, after asking the check-in question, we are not clear about what we are experiencing.

With this question, we ask the Intelligence at the heart of life to lift the clouds of our unknowing so that we can see what is going on inside us. When we ask this question we understand that whatever is happening is a part of our journey back to ourselves. It may be unpleasant, challenging, scary, overwhelming, frustrating, or simply confusing, *but it is for us.* It is bringing us necessary information that will help us to unravel the web of struggle that we are caught in. Because the question, "What is asking to be seen?" cannot be answered by the mind, it cuts through our confusion and goes straight to That Which Knows. Every time you ask this question, not only do you turn toward your experience (even though you may not be able to see anything), but you also signal the wisdom at the heart of life that you are ready for the fog to lift so that you can be present for whatever you are experiencing. You just ask, and then let it go. Even if you immediately go back into confusion, this question will be working for you underneath your reactive mind. Clarity will come in its own time and its own way.

How Can I Give This Space to Be?

If you are like me, many times on the journey back to myself, I didn't want to let whatever was happening in my life *be.* When I asked the second question, "For this moment, can I let this be here?" I often would answer it with a resounding "No!" I so wanted to believe that if I turned away from something, it would go away and leave me alone. When I finally had the courage to really look, I saw that when I tried to resist, deny, or get rid of a part of myself, it actually became stronger.

The joy I felt when I finally understood that I lessened the power of whatever I was turning away from by allowing it to exist was beyond words. So what do we do when, although we understand this truth, our resistance remains stronger than our ability to give something space to be? We go to the second open-ended question, "How can I give this space to be?" If you can feel the heart of this question, then you can feel deep relief. You do not have to figure out how to give these parts the space they need. You can ask for help in cultivating the healing of spaciousness.

How Can I Bring Compassion to This?

On the journey back to myself it also took me a while to figure out how to meet the unacceptable parts of myself with understanding and mercy. I judged and feared my experiences, so I continued to struggle. The idea of being merciful to the rejected parts of myself was completely alien to me. So when I would ask the third check-in question, "For this moment, can I touch this with compassion?" it would at times even close my heart more.

Whenever we find ourselves resisting, we can turn to the healing of the open-ended version of the third question, "For this moment, how can I bring compassion to this?" We ask this question to awaken the vast, healing regions of the heart, for that is where all true healing happens. If we love whatever comes into our lives, it loses its power over us; if we can be merciful and understanding with whatever comes into our lives, we will be free.

In the beginning, your mind may say again, "No way! I can't even begin to imagine being compassionate with myself. In fact, it is impossible." But again, the power of this question comes from the asking, which opens the door to the wisdom at the heart of life that is waiting for a question. It is important *just to keep asking!* It took years and years for your heart to completely close, locking you into the prison of struggle. It will take time to walk back out of the prison into the healing light of your open heart. Every time you ask this question, whether it feels that way or not, it takes you another step into your healing.

What Is the Way through This?

The fourth check-in question, "Right now, what do I *truly* need?" transforms into the open-ended question, "What is the way through this?" There are times on this journey back to ourselves when we don't have a clue about what is going on and our hearts are closed tighter than a drum. We may not be able to look at what we are experiencing, and we may even be resistant to acknowledging it in any way. This is when the power of the fourth open-ended question truly reveals itself. I call this the "default question" — the one you ask when you can't remember any other question. It is also the one you go to when it feels like there is nothing else to do.

I had an experience after leading one of my Hawaiian retreats that reveals how healing this question can be. At the end of the retreat, everyone drives to Kona for a few days of play and to swim with the dolphins. Since leading a retreat is wonderful but exhausting, I usually spend a day by myself to recharge and then fly home, rather than traveling with the group. One year I made the decision to go to Kona with the group, allowing no downtime in between. We didn't arrive until after dinner, and I was exhausted. When I woke up the next morning, there was not a hint of the adult within me that had just led a six-day retreat. I felt like I was four years old, and I just wanted to go home.

When I asked the first question, I could see the depth of my tiredness and the extent of my vulnerability. When I asked the second question, what I got was raging resistance to my vulnerability. I wanted to go play, and I didn't want to feel this way. In fact, I was feeling deep self-judgment for being this vulnerable. And asking the third question closed my heart even more. Needless to say, my resistance to what I was experiencing only made it worse. I had made some plans later that day and was beginning to feel a sense of dread about my commitments. When I asked what I really needed, everything was in such an uproar inside me

213

that I felt no clarity about how to bring balance back into my mind and emotions. I then asked the fourth question in an open-ended way, requesting help in showing me the way through this.

I gazed out the window for a few minutes and then noticed a mystery novel on a table across the room. It felt right to crawl back into bed and dive into the book. For the first thirty pages or so, I went back into self-judgment for being vulnerable and for being in bed in Hawaii. I also experienced fear of my commitments later on in the day. But about thirty minutes later, when I stopped reading for a few minutes and asked the check-in questions again, my heart finally opened to my weariness and vulnerability. Of course I could allow myself to be exactly where I was. I had just led a six-day retreat, so the tiredness was to be expected, and a deep peace filled me with its presence. But I didn't know what to do about the rest of the day, as I felt too tired to even get out of bed. I then asked the fourth open-ended question, "What is the way through this?" and let it go. As I went back to reading I slowly became aware of a feeling of strength coming from deep within me, and I was back in my center. I then went on to have a wonderful day of play and connection with my friends in Hawaii.

The power of the question, "What is the way through this?" is that it works for you no matter how confused and lost you are. No matter what is going on, you are not alone. The Intelligence that beats your heart and gives you breath (and is a lot smarter than you) is right there with you — even though the opposite seems true. This Intelligence is waiting for your request for help. Some people call this *surrender.* I don't like that word, because for me it carries a connotation of defeat. I like the word *open.* Through this question we *open* ourselves to the help that is always there.

Again, posing this question isn't about looking for an answer. It is about creating a space within you for an answer to come. Sometimes answers will come to you right away, and sometimes they will take time. I have lived in some questions for years, and the answers came not a moment before I was ready for them. As I look back on my journey with questions, I am stunned at the absolute perfection of this process, even though many times I have felt like I had lost my way, especially in the beginning. But it was these questions that cleared the fog and allowed me to reconnect, full of trust, with myself and with life.

Just as with the check-in questions, all four open-ended questions can be used together, or each can stand on its own. At the end of this chapter I will provide different examples of how to live in the questions. For now, just be willing to live in whatever question called to you as you read this chapter.

We can treasure hunt with questions at any time in our lives, but they are extremely powerful when our compulsions beckon to us. They are magical keys that can unlock the door of our freedom. The flavor of these questions comes from the willingness to approach ourselves with curiosity and compassion, allowing us to explore our thoughts and feelings rather than being at the mercy of them. They open the door to more and more moments of purely being present for ourselves and our lives in a fascinated and compassionate way. And most important, they connect us with the wisdom of the wellspring within us. The key is to keep on asking questions, understanding that challenges come with solutions woven into them. Our job is to pay attention, listen, and live in questions.

Other Possible Questions

The following questions have come from my own process and from the people I have worked with over the years. I have put the questions that you will most likely use as check-in questions at the top of the list, with the open-ended questions coming after. But as you will discover, some questions can be used either way. Listen to yourself, and use them in the way that works for you.

As you work with questions, the ones that are appropriate to each situation will come to you. After a while, your experiences will be accompanied by the opening of a question, and the questions you use on your treasure hunt will be creative, responsive, and a never-ending source of nourishment and wisdom. So be willing to live in questions. I still live in questions and will continue until my last breath. No, that is not right. I *am* the questions, and they constantly bring me back to a deep and nourishing connection with myself and with my life.

The First Question

The intent of asking these variations on the first question is to focus your mind on what is happening right now:

- What is the story in my head right now?
- What is happening right now?
- What are my thoughts doing right now?
- What is happening in my body?
- What do I need to notice?
- What am I resisting?
- What am I ready to see about myself and my life?
- What is the truth of my experience?

The Second Question

The intent of asking these variations on the second question is to move from reaction to response, giving whatever we are experiencing the space it needs to heal:

- For this moment can I make space for this?
- Can I accept this as a part of me?
- Can I accept this as a part of my life?
- Can I not struggle with this?
- Can I let this be so that I can be present with it?
- Can I let myself be exactly as I am?
- Can I be with this?

- How can I be with this?
- How can I accept this?
- How can I respond?
- How can I say yes to this?

The Third Question

Your intent in asking these questions is to touch whatever is present with the healing of your heart:

- What do I need to love right now?
- What do I need to love and accept about myself?
- How can I touch this with my heart?
- How can I make peace with this?
- How can I nurture myself?
- What is in need of my heart?
- What do I need to love?

The Fourth Question

The intent here is to awaken the wellspring of wisdom within us:

- What do I need to do or be that is for my highest good?
- What am I really hungry for?
- What is the kind choice here?
- What is the wise choice here?
- What is my deeper knowing?
- What is wisdom's choice?
- How can I get out of my own way?
- What is love's wisdom in this moment?

- What is the doorway through this challenge?
- How can this be healed? How do I not hate and fear this?
- Where is the humor in this?
- What shift in perspective am I ready for?
- Where is this taking me?
- What is my highest good?
- What are the treasures hidden in this experience?

Bringing Questions into Our Daily Life

As you become familiar with living in questions, you can make them your own. You may live in just one question for a while. In my life, I spent a lot of time in the beginning with just the first question. Slowly, as I learned how to be present for my experience, the second question became predominant. As I gave space to whatever I was experiencing, I began to be able to use the third question to touch it with the healing of my heart. It was only when I finally knew how to meet myself with compassion and understanding that the power of the fourth question began to reveal itself. With deep joy I finally discovered how to partner with the Intelligence at the heart of life and make wise and kind choices.

You can also blend the check-in questions and the open-ended questions in whatever way is helpful for you. You may ask the first two check-in questions and then go directly to the third open-ended question. You may ask the first open-ended question, and be able to immediately see what is going on. You then go to the fourth check-in question and hear what it is that you truly need. Listen to yourself.

The following are some examples of how to use the questions both individually and combined. I will be pulling from the list of other possible questions to show you that the most important thing to remember is the intent of each question. If you can do that, then your own individual questions will become clear to you.

Here is the scenario: You are driving home after a challenging day at work and are in a state of complete reaction. All you want to do is crawl into your compulsion.

You ask, "In this moment, what am I experiencing?" but everything inside you is in chaos, and you have no idea of the answer. You take some deep breaths, adding a pause at the end of the out- and in-breath. As you ask the question again, you are aware of feeling confused. Then it dawns on you that the answer to the first question is that what you are experiencing is confusion! You then go to the second question, "For this moment, can I let this confusion be here?"

This question reminds you that if you fight with it, it will only get worse and will probably make your compulsion look very interesting. If you can give it space, then it can move through you rather than you getting lost in it. The second time you ask if you can let this be, a yes comes up inside of you — "Yes, I can let this be for just this moment."

This opens up a space inside you where you can *relate* to what is going on rather than being *lost in it*. Immediately your attention is drawn to a knot of tension inside you. Knowing that this tension is created by some feelings that are burbling within you, you ask a variation of the first question, "Right now, what am I feeling?"

As you keep your attention on the knot of tension, it reveals itself as fear. You hear the voices that go along with this fear saying, "I am afraid that if I don't do my job right, I will be fired."

You immediately ask, "For this moment, can I touch this with compassion?" This question opens your heart, and you now can touch this scared part of yourself with understanding and mercy. You tell this feeling that you are listening and that it is okay that it is here.

You then go to the fourth question, "Right now, what do I *truly* need?" A desire to be compulsive flits through your mind. But because you have been willing to turn toward yourself rather than away, it is clear to you that no matter how much you want to act on your compulsion, it will only make you feel better temporarily, and, in the long run, it will make you feel worse.

When you ask the question again, you remember that the wellspring of wisdom within you waits for the opening of a question. A few stoplights later, you become clear that tomorrow you want to review the report you were concerned about so that you can discuss it with your boss. You will then be more familiar with it and know where your boss stands on the issues. This starts to unravel the knot of fear, but visions of your compulsion are still lingering.

When you ask again, "Right now, what do I *truly* need?" you feel that you need to do something that will allow you to stay connected to yourself in a comforting and balanced way. You consider the possibility of buying the paper, going to a coffee house, and having a latte while you read. "No," says your wisdom. "It would feel better to be with somebody I am comfortable with and do something fun." So you call a good friend and make plans to see an upbeat movie together.

But suppose you get all the way to the fourth question, "Right now, what do I *truly* need?" and you find resistance again. "All I want is my compulsion," demands the scared part of you. Reaction begins to cloud your mind again, so you go back to the first question, "In this moment, what am I experiencing?" You feel the craving for your compulsion deep inside you, and you speak the truth of this to yourself.

You realize that if you fight this craving, it will only make it worse. You then ask, "For this moment, can I let this craving be?" Because you truly understand that if you resist it, it will only get worse, the answer is, "Yes." In this spaciousness, the cravings calm down. You take some deep breaths, gently and mercifully breathing into the tightness inside you. Your mind is now clear enough that you can ask again, "What do I *truly* need?" This question opens your heart and reminds you that what you truly need is a healing connection with yourself. You bring your hand over your heart and tell yourself that you understand that it was a very challenging day and that you are here for yourself right now. You keep your hand over your heart all the way home, and, as your reactions fall away, you have a wonderful evening.

Suppose you ask the question, "In this moment, what am I experiencing?" and nothing inside you wants to look at, let alone listen to, what is going on. In fact, the question fans the flame of anger within you, and you feel not the slightest willingness to explore your inner experience. All you want is to yield to your compulsion.

Immediately you go to the fourth open-ended question, "What is the way through this?" You then let that question go, allowing it to work for you. This doesn't stop the wave of compulsion, but that is okay. It is a shorter wave than usual because very quickly it becomes clear to you that being compulsive isn't helping you feel better.

While lying in bed later that night, feeling uncomfortable from the effects of having been compulsive, the first question pops into your mind: "In this moment, what am I experiencing?" At first glance all you feel is a thick fog. But you stay with the question, knowing that it will clear up the fog so you can see and be with what is going on within you. As the fog lifts, you feel the overall feeling of discomfort in your body.

When you ask, "For this moment, can I let this be here?" your immediate response is, "No! I screwed up again." But that contraction is so painful that you are willing to ask this question in an open-ended way: "For this moment, *how* can I let myself be exactly as I am?" (a variation on the second open-ended question).

This question reminds you that if you struggle with where you are, it only makes things worse. If you allow it to be and pay attention, things will lighten up, and you will learn something. As you take some deep breaths, it comes to you that you weren't compulsive because you are weak-willed or defective. Instead, there is something inside you that you don't yet know how to take care of in any other way. You also remember that if you focus on what is going on inside you right now, without judging yourself, you will see more clearly that the price you pay for your compulsion is just too high.

So you ask the first open-ended question: "What is asking to be seen?" You are asking for clarity from the deep Intelligence that is always with you. As you bring your attention into your body and begin to explore exactly what you are experiencing, you write down on a pad of paper everything you discover — the ball of dread in your belly, the pounding of your heart, the tight shoulders, the acid stomach, and the empty hole deep within you.

You then ask, "Right now, what do I *truly* need?" You feel compelled to open this book to a random page and read whatever you see first. What you read opens your heart to yourself again, and your self-judgment lightens. As you turn out the lights, you ask for help through the fourth open-ended question, "What is the way through this?" knowing that it will work for you while you are asleep.

The art of asking questions is exactly that — an art. A pianist doesn't play Mozart after a few lessons, and you won't master the art of treasure hunting with these questions overnight. Be willing to ask questions all the time, even when you don't want to know what you are experiencing, when you can't open to what you are experiencing, and even when you don't trust that the questions will make any difference. Just keep asking, and the questions will support you in ways you cannot even imagine. Know also that it doesn't matter if you can only stay in the space of a question for a moment or two. Just like a small pebble thrown into a huge lake, its ripples eventually make it all the way to the shore. One question sets things in motion, moving you farther down the path of awakening.

Let us now explore how we can use these questions to transform our experience, first through taking them into the sensations in our bodies, then our feelings, and finally our compulsions.

Core Ideas

- The power of questions lies in the questions themselves!

- Check-in questions allow us to meet and transform whatever we are experiencing.

- The quickest and most powerful way to dissolve your struggles is to let them be.

- Asking these questions awakens your inner wellspring, making it easier over time to hear exactly what will bring peace into your life.

- In asking open-ended questions we are not looking for answers. Instead we are opening ourselves so that answers can come to us from the deepest and wisest parts of ourselves.

- The beauty of asking open-ended questions, allowing the Universe to answer rather than relying on our own limited intelligence, is that we don't just *get* an answer. We *become* the answer itself.

- The art of trusting that the Intelligence of the Universe will answer our questions comes to each of us in its own time and its own way.

- The core healing that compulsions bring you is the knowing that no matter what is going on, you are not alone. The Intelligence that beats your heart and gives you breath (and is a lot smarter than you) is right there with you, waiting for your request for help.

- Be willing to ask questions all the time, even when you don't want to know what you are experiencing, when you can't open to what you are experiencing, and even when you don't trust that the questions will make any difference. Just keep asking, and the questions will support you in ways you cannot even imagine.

Chapter 13

....

TREASURE HUNTING WITH

Sensations

We have arrived at the heart of the matter, where healing and being healed by our compulsions occurs — we are ready to go treasure hunting. As we clearly see by now, our readiness to heal and be healed is signaled by our increased ability to shine the light of our attention on whatever we are experiencing as we are experiencing it, our willingness to allow whatever is there to be there, and the power of our hearts to transform whatever sensations, thoughts, and feelings are asking for our attention. Through our compassionate curiosity, old patterns dissolve back into the aliveness that we truly are. Our attention is then freed from reaction so that we can listen to the deep knowing within us. In this listening, we can make wise and skillful choices that allow us to open again to the joy of being fully connected to ourselves and to our lives.

The more skilled you become at acknowledging your experience exactly as it is, the easier it will be to see and then to let go of layers upon layers of old thoughts, feelings, and patterns that used to drive your actions. You can also find the treasures that lie buried within every experience of your life, no matter how confusing or painful.

The Wise Teacher of Our Bodies

We have all been well taught not to feel what we feel, distracting ourselves instead. We have become so good at drowning out the signals from our inner world that it's no wonder that we are compulsive a good deal of the time.

So how do we gather the inner treasures that are waiting for us? It may seem impossible at first glance, but I assure you it is simpler and safer than you can imagine. We will begin by exploring the deep wisdom of our bodies, and then we will use the four questions discussed in the last chapter to explore our sensations. The sensations we find in our bodies can be our training ground for learning how to notice what we are experiencing and then to transform our experience through spaciousness and mercy. In the beginning, seeing what is happening in our heads can be a bit difficult, for the thoughts that run us can be very seductive. And the feelings that ensnare us can either be very elusive or very intense. We get so identified with them that we become lost in a story *about* what we are experiencing rather than *experiencing* it.

The easiest place to learn how to see and be real about what we are experiencing is to focus on our sensations. Every moment of our lives a river of sensations flows through our bodies. And these sensations are not just random experiences. Our bodies are speaking to us all the time from a depth of wisdom beyond our comprehension. In fact, the body is one of the wisest and dearest friends we will ever have.

The human body has been around for a very long time, and it has developed the capacity to survive by being highly tuned into exactly what is going on. While our heads are spinning all sorts of tales about what we *should be* experiencing, the body will never lie. If somebody has made us angry, even if we try to hide our anger, even if we tell ourselves that we aren't angry, our body will raise our heartbeat and tighten our stomach. It tells us the truth of the situation.

To acknowledge the truth of what is happening in our bodies we need to understand the difference between basic sensations and sensations that are fueled by feelings. Basic sensations are like a tickle in our throat, the coolness of the air, the pressure of a chair against our thighs. These sensations are not generated by feelings. There is another level of sensations that are generated by feelings — that lump in your throat, the butterflies in your stomach, the empty feeling in your belly. In other words, feelings generate sensations in your body. Think of what happens in your body when you are excited or afraid, and you will know what I mean.

At the beginning, instead of looking for the feelings that fuel our compulsions we simply focus on our sensations, for our bodies can teach us how to be simply present with what we are experiencing. Over the years I have seen people develop the ability to be present for themselves just by paying attention to their sensations, and they are delighted. "I can feel myself again," they often say. As we develop our ability to be present through our sensations, the feelings that generate many of them will begin to reveal themselves — a process we'll explore in depth in the next chapter. That lump in the throat begins to reveal a deep sadness. That tightness in the chest reveals anxiety. That knot in the belly reveals a deep fear. And rather than reacting to these emotions, we can be present for them in the same way we learned how to be present for jitters in the legs, a deep hunger in the stomach, tension in the neck.

Using the Four Questions to Check into Our Bodies

If you are like most people, you aren't used to checking into your body. At the beginning it can be helpful to focus on the following three areas where feelings and their corresponding sensations most often exist:

1. *The head, neck, and shoulders.* Look for raised shoulders, clenched jaws, dizziness, throbbing temples, pressure behind the eyes, shooting pains along the side of the head, a dull ache in

the forehead, a sore tongue, burning between the shoulder blades, a lump of happiness or sadness in the throat, and so on.

2. *The chest.* Look for pressure on the chest, out-of-control excitement, a tight band of tension that makes it hard to breathe, sharp pains, shallow breathing, a racing pulse, heart palpitations, or overall thrills.

3. *The belly.* Look for the excitement of butterflies or fists of tension in the stomach, tight bands across the lower pelvic region, unbounded energy, sharp pains, explosive pressure, sexual excitement, empty holes right around the belly button, sinking sensations, and queasiness.

As you explore these areas, also bring your attention into your backside. We hide so many of our unacceptable parts of ourselves "behind" us and they show up as tightened muscles, burning aches, and throbbing pains in various areas in our back. Let us now explore bringing the four questions to all these myriad sensations.

In This Moment, What Am I Experiencing?

Curiosity is about turning the mind into a flashlight and shining it on what is truly happening inside us at any given moment. It turns our attention away from *what was* and *what will be* and leads us to look at *what is happening right now.* And curiosity is what this main question, "In this moment, what am I experiencing?" and its open-ended version, "What is asking to be seen?" are all about. This question also allows us to dissolve whatever is keeping us from being fully open to life. As we develop the capacity to be present for what we are experiencing in our body, we can dissolve many of the sensations that used to bring discomfort and disconnection just through the light of our attention. I have known deep contraction in my body, especially in my neck and belly. Using this question, I can now stay current with these old patterns of contracting and let them go before they take over my body again.

Let us practice taking the check-in question into our sensations.

Exercise

After you read this exercise, close your eyes and take a few deep breaths to focus your mind. As you settle in, add a short pause at the end of the in-breath and at the end of the out-breath. As your mind quiets down, bring your attention to your body and ask the question, "In this moment, what am I experiencing?"

Be curious about your sensations, allowing your attention to be like a flashlight searching your body. Check in with the three main areas, for somewhere in your body resides a pocket of strong sensations. You don't need to make a big production out of this. Stay in each area for no more than a breath or two, noticing what's happening. When you have touched on all three areas, go back to the place that felt the most constricted and allow your attention to rest there for a short while. As you allow your attention and your sensations to meet, what you are experiencing will become clearer.

Don't rush this. Allow the sensations to come to you. Then speak the truth to yourself about what is happening there. Some of the things you may be able to name are tingles, warmth, coolness, tightness, tenderness, pressure, restlessness, agitation, sharp pain, throbbing, tickles, aches. Whenever your attention wanders away, gently bring it back again to your sensations. Stay with them as long as you can, even if it is just for a moment or two. If you want to stay there longer, keep speaking the truth of your experience to yourself. This will deepen your ability to relate to what you are exploring rather than getting lost in it.

Be patient. Know that even though you may not be able to feel it, the tension is beginning to release under the light of your attention. It may not dramatically dissolve at first, for the laser beam of your attention is not yet strong enough. But know that the more you cultivate the ability and the willingness to be present for what is happening in your body, the more your tension will dissolve under the light of your attention.

This is a good practice to do every morning for a few minutes before you get out of bed. You can also do it whenever there's a pause in your life — when you're on hold for an appointment, standing in line, waiting for your food to arrive. You may find that a sensation, rather than letting go, seems to become stronger through your focused attention. Especially at the beginning of the journey back to yourself, this is very normal. This does not mean that your attention is amplifying anything. Rather, since you have lifted the fog of your resistance, you are more aware of what is going on. And even though it may seem like your experience is being amplified, the opposite is true. The light of your attention is beginning to work its magic on this old pattern.

In contrast, you may discover that when you are invited to pay attention to what you're experiencing in your body, you can't feel a thing. This is also very common. We have been so educated out of our bodies and so trained to deny our immediate experience that when we first become curious about it, all we may discover is fog or a blank wall. You may even feel quite a bit of resistance to experiencing your sensations at all. Don't be dismayed. This is very normal at the beginning. That is where the open-ended questions come in. You can ask the first one, "What is asking to be seen?" and then let it go. It will work its magic from underneath your everyday consciousness, clearing the fog and the resistance until, with simple clarity, you can discover what you are experiencing.

The ability to bring your attention to your immediate experience and then to speak the truth to yourself about what you are experiencing is what will eventually help you to unravel the tangled web of compulsions. It may take a while for you to fully understand the phenomenal power of what we are exploring here, for the mind deeply believes in fixing, changing, and dominating. But these compensatory behaviors are nothing in comparison to the power of bringing the light of our focused and compassionate attention to our immediate experience.

When people I work with learn how to pay attention to their experience, they are often stunned by how completely they have been able to pull the wool over their own eyes — stunned but delighted, for it is such a relief to finally be real about what is going on. As we move from reaction to response, meeting ourselves as we are, our focused attention acts like a laser beam, transforming whatever it rests on. And many of the sensations, feelings, and thoughts that fuel our compulsions will dissolve under the light of this attention. The more we do this, the quicker our old patterns will melt away. If they don't, we can then move on to one or all three of the processing questions.

For This Moment, Can I Let This Be Here?

This first of the three processing questions is about cultivating spaciousness. "For this moment, can I let this be here?" and its open-ended version, "How can I give this the space to be?" are all about allowing ourselves to be exactly where we are. To learn the power of letting something be is such an important step in our healing, for we are deeply programmed in its opposite — fight or flight. Either we struggle with unwanted experiences, or we run away from them as fast as we can.

One of the best places to see the power of giving our experience space is in our bodies. Take a cramp in your leg, for example. If you tighten down, it hurts more. If you move toward the experience instead, allowing the calf muscles to relax, the pain moves through like an ocean wave rather than a knife tearing up your leg. Giving your sensations space also gives you room to explore them. Imagine holding something unpleasant in your hand, clenching and wringing it thoroughly to crush it out of existence. At first, you can't see what you are resisting. Then, when you open your hand, it is still there (only in a more mutilated state!). But if you open your hand fully, you can now see what you were contracting around. You can become familiar with it, exploring its depth and breadth, gathering the information you need to heal. And when it is time, with just a subtle tilt of your hand, you can let it go.

With the first question, we learned how to use the light of our attention to recognize and transform a pocket of tension. If tension persists, we are now learning to give it permission to be there, for it is in spaciousness that sensations, thoughts, and feelings move through us. Let us explore how to cultivate spaciousness around our sensations.

Exercise

After you read this exercise, close your eyes and take a few deep breaths to focus your mind. As you settle in, add a short pause at the end of the in-breath and at the end of the out-breath. As your mind quiets down, bring your attention to the pocket of tension you were working with before. On the next in-breath imagine that you are drawing air into a balloon that is at the center of the tension. Gently open up this pocket of tension with your breath. Then on the out-breath, you say one long *ahhhhh* out loud, and allow your body to let go of the tension. The in-breath opens the tightness of reaction that usually surrounds the tension in our bodies. The out-breath invites that tension to release.

Breathe this Balloon Breath as many times as you want, then go back to your normal breath. Keeping your focus on the area of tension, ask the second question: "For this moment, can I let this be here?" Let that question soften any remaining resistance so that you can fully be present for whatever is there. Just asking this question signals that you are choosing to respond rather than to react. Given enough space, this pocket of tension will feel permission to let go. The release may feel like a physical opening or a warmth that comes from the locked energy being released. Sometimes this wave of letting go will expand and fill your whole body with cascading warmth and joy. Even if you feel nothing dissolve, your attention is laying the foundation for future releases.

If nothing lets go, you can move to the open-ended version of the second question, "How can I give this space to be?" Another variation of that question is, "How can I not struggle with this?" Every time you ask an open-ended question, wisdom will come into the vacuum that you have created. This wisdom will awaken your heart, allowing you to live in the healing of response rather than in the struggle of reaction. If you find yourself closing in reaction, ask the fourth open-ended question, the "default question": "What is the way through this?" Then let that question go; it will work for you,

> even though it may seem that nothing is happening. Know also that
> just asking open-ended questions is very healing.

In This Moment, Can I Touch This with Compassion?

The intent of this third question is to tap us into the phenomenal power of compassion. It invites us to meet ourselves with the healing of our hearts. Before I learned about compassion, there was always an undercurrent of harshness in my response to the unpleasantness in my body. "Oh, you again," my mind would say. And then from somewhere in the depths a knife of self-judgment would surface: "Look at you, you overly sensitive drama queen."

Needless to say, these voices did absolutely nothing to calm my body. In fact, they usually made it worse. But over the years, the power of being merciful with myself slowly began to creep in underneath all my harshness and judgment. This ability to bring the light of our hearts to our immediate experience is embodied in the third question, "In this moment, can I touch this with compassion?" and its open-ended version, "How can I bring compassion to this?"

I can still remember the first time when I was not feeling well and rather than resisting what I was experiencing, I felt compassion. Something that Stephen Levine once said crept lightly into my consciousness: "Treat yourself as if you were your only child." Reflecting on this simple statement, I asked myself what I would do if I were a child feeling the same things I was feeling. Of course, my heart opened and I drew that imaginary child into my heart.

I then turned the light of compassion toward myself, and, wonder of wonders, I felt such tenderness. And of course doing this calmed down whatever I was experiencing and showed me how deeply starved I was for my own mercy. From that time on, I began to cultivate compassion for everything I resisted. If I couldn't muster any, I would immediately ask myself what I would do with a child experiencing the same thing I was going through. This little trick showed me what I was truly longing for, and I was then able to give it to myself.

Let us now continue our exploration. First we used the light of our attention to recognize and then dissolve the tension in our bodies. Then we focused on the power of giving our immediate experience the space to *be*. Let us now add the willingness to touch it with our hearts.

Exercise

After you read this exercise, close your eyes and take a few deep breaths to focus your mind. As you settle in, add a short pause at the end of the in-breath and at the end of the out-breath. As your mind quiets down, bring your attention to the middle of your chest and begin to breathe through your heart. If you have never done this before, picture a little nose on your chest and imagine your breath coming in and out of that nose. As you let your attention rest there, you can begin to feel your heart center being touched and opened by the intention of this breath. Now open the field of your attention and find a sensation in your body that you consider mildly unpleasant. If nothing is there right now, imagine an experience from the past — a headache, queasiness, twitchy legs. As you continue to breathe through your heart, ask the third question, "For this moment, can I touch this with compassion?" Then on the out-breath send this heart energy to the area in your body you are working with, and surround this experience with the healing of compassion. Remember, just like you, these unpleasant sensations respond to kindness and mercy.

If your heart doesn't begin to open, imagine a child who is experiencing what you are and imagine being tender with him. Then allow your body to feel the benefits of this compassion for someone else. And on your out-breath, send this compassion to whatever part of your body you are working with.

If your heart still does not open, go to the open-ended version of this question, "How can I bring compassion to this?" and know that this question will be working for you whether or not you notice anything.

All the parts of your body that you have formerly reacted to long for the healing of your compassion. This place of touching ourselves with our hearts is where all lasting healing happens. For the heart merges all opposites, all extremes, all challenges of our lives into the healing of mercy.

Right Now, What Do I Truly Need?

Everything we are exploring here is about clearing up enough of our old patterns so that we can listen to our own deep knowing. In fact, it could be said that compulsions are given to us because we cannot control them. And coming across something we cannot fix opens us to the possibility of creating a partnership with the wellspring of deep knowing within us, which always leads us toward our highest good.

You can clear the pathway to your own deep knowing through working with the fourth question, "Right now, what do I *truly* need?" Remember, we aren't trying to figure out the answers to this question. Rather, we ask it to attune to the inner wellspring that knows the most empowering thing to do in any situation. Then the answers, rather than coming from our heads, come from *within us.* Rather than struggling to apply mind-created answers in our lives, we find ourselves *living the answers.* We can also ask this question directly of the sensations we are noticing in our bodies by saying, "What do *you* truly need?" Many of our challenging sensations such as headaches, burning stomachs, tricky backs, aching feet, and heart palpitations, if asked, will reveal the next step we need to take to bring our bodies back into balance.

The mind has a tendency to become frustrated when it doesn't get an immediate answer. Be patient. It is much more powerful to *live* answers than to *get* them. And know that the more you use this question, the quicker and clearer the answers will be. At the beginning this may not happen right away, so you can then ask the open-ended version of this question, "What is the way through this?" Remember, it isn't necessary to receive immediate wisdom. Just the power of the question sets things in motion.

You may get this far only to be pulled back into the vortex of reaction when you ask for clarity in what you *truly* need. Don't worry; that is a part of the awakening process. We are like babies learning how to walk. We will fall down over and over again in our quest to understand and cultivate this partnership with our inner wisdom. Know that this question is awakening your deep wisdom, and just like a peach ripens from a hard green nugget to a round, golden globe, you too are being ripened into the goldenness of true partnership.

You may even get a clear answer but not want to act on it. The pull to stay caught in reaction may be much stronger than the desire to act wisely. At times that is to be expected; we will explore what to do in this situation in chapter 15. Until then, know that every time you ask this question, you are activating the wisdom within you that knows how to make kind and skillful choices.

Let us now complete this exploration by learning to listen to our inner wellspring. As with the other questions, the fourth question can be used following the other three questions or all on its own. In fact, "Right now, what do I *truly* need?" is a very skillful question to work with even when there's nothing much going on.

Exercise

After you read this exercise, close your eyes and take a few deep breaths to focus your mind. As you settle in, add a short pause at the end of the in-breath and at the end of the out-breath. Now that you have brought spaciousness and mercy to your experience, your ability to hear your own wisdom has become stronger. Bring to mind the sensation you have been exploring and ask yourself, "Right now, what do I truly need to bring this back into balance?" Listen to the deep part of you that knows what needs to be done to bring this sensation back into balance. If nothing becomes clear, know that this question is waking up your wellspring within and you will live the answers at the appropriate time.

When asking the fourth question, we need to understand that no matter where we are and no matter what is happening, our deepest need is connection with the fullness of life, right here, right now. So it can be very healing when we are listening to what we *truly* need to pause before we take the next step in our lives and give ourselves the gift of being fully present with life. This is about focusing on something bigger than whatever has been capturing our attention within us. Because the mind loves to attach to the narrow world of trying to figure out and "do" life, it can be very powerful to learn that a lot more is going on in life than the struggles we get lost in and that we do have a choice about where we are going to place our attention. We *can* place it again on the pure gift of life, right here, right now. For this is the only moment when life is truly happening.

It isn't always easy to pull our attention away from struggle and place it again in the immediacy of life — especially at the beginning of our awakening. Some of the old patterns in our bodies, minds, and hearts can feel all-encompassing. But they aren't. Pain in our body, a deep emotion, a very seductive mental pattern: these are just a part of the story that we took on when we were little — a story *about* life rather than the real thing. If we broaden our focus to include the fullness of this moment, we see that life is about so much more than this story in our heads. We then become bigger than what we are experiencing. *We are not our thoughts, our feelings, or the sensations in our bodies. We are that which can see them!* The more we pay attention, the clearer this truth will be, and the clearer it becomes, the more freedom we will know.

Rather than paying attention to our struggles, we can broaden our focus to include the whole body, discovering many areas that are doing just fine. We are alive; our heart is beating; our breath is rising and falling; tingles of aliveness are everywhere. We can open even further, reconnecting with the fullness of life right here, right now — the music of sound as it swells and recedes all around us, the variations of light that surround us, the amazing gift of life.

Let us now practice bringing our attention back onto life.

Exercise

After you read this exercise, close your eyes and take a few deep breaths to focus your mind. As you settle in, add a short pause at the end of the in-breath and at the end of the out-breath. Now place your attention on the sounds of life around you — the music of birds, the hum of voices, the sound of cars. As you relish them for a few moments, recognize that you are listening to your life the moment it appears out of mystery! All the millions of moments of your life have brought you here to this moment, and this is the only one that matters. When your attention drifts off, bring it back to the sounds and notice the big difference between being caught in the narrow world of your mind and being present with life the moment it appears out of mystery. When you are ready, open your eyes.

In time these questions will become automatic. When you turn toward your experience, your curiosity will immediately be drawn to the area that needs your undivided attention. In just two or three breaths you give it the attention that it needs to open again, transforming it with your heart. You will then see clearly what needs to be done to bring balance into your life. The energy that was formerly caught in tension is now freed back into the field of being, and you are available again for the fullness of life.

Enhancing the Questions with Our Breath

As we bring our attention into the sensations in our bodies we can greatly enhance the power of these questions through working with the breath. As we explored in chapter 9, opening to our breath is an invaluable skill to use in our journey back to ourselves. The wonderful thing about this skill is that it can be as simple as taking just one deep breath. When we are caught in the middle of an inner storm, taking one conscious breath can help immensely to calm things down.

We can also do many other things with our breath. We can simply add a short pause at the end of the in-breath and at the end of the out-breath. These pauses activate our parasympathetic nervous system, the part of us that calms us down. They also signal our mind that we are moving into a deeper level of consciousness. We can breathe into the holdings in our bodies, gently opening the constriction from the inside with our breath. We can breathe very fast, changing the biochemistry of our body and moving any tension right through us. We can also add a few deep breaths to an activity we do many times throughout the day — washing our hands, walking down a hallway at work, waiting at stoplights, and so forth. Doing this keeps us attuned to the great river of breath and keeps us present. If you want to work with other breath techniques, reread chapter 9. The most important thing is to keep bringing your attention back to your breath. Notice that when you are caught in the stories in your head, your breath is usually shallow. Just noticing this allows your breath to become an exquisite biofeedback system alerting you very early on when an old pattern is taking over. And when you can, release the pattern by taking one deep breath.

When There Is No Release

You will come across constrictions in your body that won't immediately release, even in the light of your open and focused attention. Know that your willingness to be present with them — even if it is for just a moment or two — and to ask the questions is taking you down the pathway of your healing. In addition, here are two simple ways to keep things opening:

Ask the Default Question

This technique is short and sweet. If you are stuck and don't know what to do, don't have any inclination to do anything, and in fact want to just escape your experience, before you do anything, pause for just a moment and ask the fourth open-ended question, "What is the way through this?"

In my life, this question has come down to two words — "show me." I say these words multiple times a day, not only to remind myself that something much smarter than I is in charge, but also to build a partnership with this wisdom at the heart of life. Know that every time you ask this question, you are signaling the wisdom at the heart of life that you are ready and willing to know full partnership.

Get Moving

The second thing we can do when we feel caught with no way out is to *move.* Movement is such a powerful healing force. Watch the wind dance. Watch water as it cascades and crashes, laps and whirls. All life is in constant motion. And what do we do with a baby who is fussing? We move her! We rock and walk and swing and jiggle. And usually this calms her down. The pockets of tension in your body want to move too. Remember, whenever you are caught in an old pattern in your body, your mind, or your emotions, that these patterns are just energy that has become restricted.

Movement can be as simple as taking deep breaths, as healing as cleaning the house, or as liberating as getting outside. It can be as wild as putting on some music and dancing, or it can be as gentle as lying on your side and rocking your body back and forth with your hand over your heart. When you feel contracted, little movements can go a long way toward opening you back up. After all, the mighty Columbia River starts as a rivulet flowing from a lofty mountain.

An experience from my life shows how healing it is to get physically moving. One morning I woke up in despair. It was a very busy period, and at the same time a dear friend of mine was dying. My mind was tired enough that I didn't have the energy it takes to meet the overwhelm I was feeling. And yet I knew that in order to not be engulfed by my despair, I needed to respond to it rather than react. I considered staying in bed for a while, cuddling with myself. Sometimes that is very appropriate, but my wisest part recognized that on this occasion it would cause me to freeze even more.

As I listened to my body, I knew it wanted to move. But this despair, being very contracted and very young, wanted to stay frozen just as a deer freezes in the presence of a hunter. I was split: 49.999 percent of me wanted to stay behind the prison walls of despair, but 50.001 percent of me wanted to open again. With resistance screaming in my head, I got on my exercise bike and began to peddle. For the first two minutes I wanted to stop and hide. Then my energy began to move. Oh, the bliss of that ride! Waves of energy flowed from the top of my head to the tips of my toes. And the joy that came from having opened rather than closing up was palpable.

Running, massaging, dancing, singing, hiking, gardening, playing with your dog, doing yoga, stretching: all these move your energy. It is amazing what a ten-minute walk will do to move things through, leaving you more refreshed and more connected with yourself. If you can remind yourself, especially when you are really tight and uneasy, that movement changes your body, your mind, and your heart, you can dramatically shift your experience. For simplicity, let us explore some techniques that can be used right where you are. One of my favorite ways to invite a pocket of tension in my body to move again is to exaggerate it. On an in-breath, I tighten my whole body, and as I breathe out, I let it all go, melting back into life. You can do this with individual parts of your body that are tight, and you can do it with your whole body. The reason this works so well is that muscles literally cannot hold on to tension that is exaggerated.

If your body needs more than just a few deep breaths along with some exaggeration, stand with your feet at least two feet apart. Then put your hands together and raise them above your head. Then, just as if you were chopping wood, very forcefully bring your hands down between your legs as you say as loud as you can, "Ha!" Do this a number of times, allowing your "Ha!" to come from as deep in your body as you can. This "Ha!" Breath really gets things going.

Another way to open ourselves is to use a very powerful breathing technique called the Breath of Fire. In this exercise your main focus is on the out-breath. Try it after reading the following paragraph:

Exercise

Breathing through your nose, on your next out-breath, pull your belly in with a snap, forcing the air out of your lungs. Then relax your belly and let the in-breath come naturally. Then snap your belly again to begin the out-breath and relax the belly on the in-breath. After a few practice breaths, begin to speed up the pace of your breath so that it sounds as if you were a train engine going faster and faster. Remember, the power of this breath comes from focusing on the out-breath. Be careful with this breath. Most people are not used to getting this oxygenated, and it can make them dizzy. If you become light-headed, stop for a few moments.

Singing is also a great way to get energy moving again. Sing favorite songs, silly songs, inspirational songs. You don't even need to sing or even to carry a tune. You can chant a vowel sound like *ah,* letting it resonate in your chest and opening any constriction there. You can chant the sound *oh,* giving it a deep tone so that it can open your belly. The sound of the vowel *i* that moves into *eee,* causing your neck muscles to pop out, opens your neck and throat. The sound of *ay* or *eee* chanted in the higher ranges can open your head.

However you choose to move your energy, it is important to do this *after* you have brought the light of your attention to whatever you are experiencing — even if it is just for a few moments and even if you don't recognize what is going on. You can make tension dissolve with these techniques, but if you aren't cultivating the willingness to be present with it — at least for a moment or two — it will keep coming back until it is fully transformed.

And if you can't move — either your body doesn't allow it or you're just too contracted — smile. It is amazing what a smile will do to your flow of energy. Smiling helps you to accept that on some level this is no big deal. After all, it is just trapped energy, a block in the flow of aliveness that you truly are.

If none of these techniques works, it just means that the pattern is not ready to let go. Most likely the feeling that is showing up as these sensations needs your attention too. In the next chapter we will explore how to use the light of our attention to transform even the deepest of feelings. For now, know that *paying attention to the sensations in your body makes it safe for these feelings to reveal themselves.*

Check in throughout the Day

To practice bringing the four questions into your immediate experience keeps you up-to-date with yourself. *As you do quick check-ins throughout the day, you train your mind to be curious about what is happening right now rather than always trying to change what is.* You can take a breath and ask the question, "In this moment, what am I experiencing?" while watching TV, at a business meeting, or while riding on a bus. You can ask the question when you are brushing your teeth, waiting for the doctor, driving your car, getting a massage, sitting at the theater, or falling asleep at night.

Then you can speak the truth to yourself about what is happening. Every time you name what you are experiencing, you have created more space around it, for in that moment *you are relating to it rather than being lost in it.* And if your experience is not transformed through the light of your attention, then work with the three processing questions. As you learn how to be present in a spacious way with the sensations in your body, you can then take your developing attention into the feelings that fuel your compulsions. Let us turn to that now.

Core Ideas

- The sensations we find in our bodies can be our training ground for learning how to notice what we are experiencing and then to transform our experience through spaciousness and mercy.

- Feelings generate sensations in your body — that lump in your throat, the butterflies in your stomach, the empty experience in your belly.

- As we move from reaction to response, meeting ourselves as we are, our focused attention acts like a laser beam, transforming whatever it rests on. And many of the sensations, feelings, and thoughts that fuel our compulsions will dissolve under the light of this attention.

- Our bodies are one of the best places to relearn the art of allowing our experience to be.

- All the parts of your body that you formerly reacted to long for the healing of your compassion. This place of touching ourselves with our hearts is where all lasting healing happens.

- Know that every time you ask your sensations what they *truly* need, you are activating the wisdom within you that knows how to make kind and skillful choices.

- Rather than paying attention only to our struggles, we can broaden our focus to include the whole body, discovering many areas that are doing just fine. We can open even further, reconnecting with the fullness of life right here, right now.

- You will come across constrictions in your body that won't immediately release, even in the light of your open and focused attention. Know that your willingness to be present with them and to ask the questions — even if it is for just a moment or two — is taking you down the pathway of your healing.

Chapter 14

TREASURE HUNTING WITH

Feelings

We have been exploring the art of tuning into our immediate experience so that it can be transformed through the healing light of our compassionate attention. For a while, working with physical sensations may be all we can do. That is enough. *Don't rush this process.* Just asking yourself, "In this moment, what am I experiencing?" and then being present for a lump in your throat or a knot in your stomach is a step on the path back to yourself. And if you can't let it be, that is okay too. Just the willingness to ask if you can let it be will loosen the constriction. Also, it may be too much even to contemplate touching your experience with your heart. Ask how you can touch this with compassion, and then let the healing of mercy come in its own time and its own way. And know that even if nothing becomes clear when you ask the question "Right now, what do I *truly* need?" the question is still working for you underneath your everyday awareness, awakening your own deep knowing.

As you strengthen your capacity to be present by paying attention to your body, there comes a time to bring this level of compassionate attention into the feelings that are showing up as many of the sensations in your body — the happiness that creates a lump in your throat, the sadness that feels like an elephant sitting on your chest, the out-of-control exuberance throughout your body, the anger that shows up as a knot in your stomach, the fear that tightens your belly.

We need to understand two things before we begin treasure hunting with our feelings. First, each of us is a mixture of dark and light. We need both polarities to exist. We are made up of the uplifting and lighter energies such as joy, faith, and humility. We also carry the heavier and darker energies such as judgment, fear, anger, and sorrow. Not only is it normal to have both positive and negative traits, it is necessary! We are created out of dark and light, remembering and forgetting, strengths and weaknesses.

Lynn Andrews summed up this truth beautifully in her book *Jaguar Woman:* "If you look at something carefully... you will always be able to see the dark side too. And yet we choose never to look into the shadows....Understand that it is what you choose not to observe in your life that controls your life....Everything begins with a circle of motion; without positive and negative poles there would be no movement, no creation....Without the dark side your beauty would not exist. Don't be afraid to look at both sides. You need them both...honor all as part of the Great Spirit."[1]

Our lives are also a dance of dark and light. We were sold a debilitating bill of goods when we were young — the whole idea that we are here to live happily ever after. The full spectrum of life includes both the easy *and* the difficult. We are all familiar with the old saying "Into every life a little rain will fall." Most of us don't just experience gentle showers. We also know thunderstorms and windstorms and midwinter gales that rip the limbs off of the trees of our souls. But rain makes things grow, and windstorms open spaces in the forest of our hearts, allowing for new growth to appear.

We also have sweet summer mornings when the air is full of rich, intoxicating smells and the sparkle of dew is more breathtaking than the most exquisite jewel. But the ease of summer inside us inevitably moves into the storms of winter again, and if we try to hold on, it only causes suffering. Just like the seasons, life will constantly rock back and forth between the pleasant and the unpleasant. Our peace comes when we realize that our lives will continually move through the full spectrum. If we can learn to ride the waves, we can tap into a deeper, trust-filled peace.

Thich Nhat Hanh, the Vietnamese monk and activist who was nominated for a Nobel Peace Prize by Martin Luther King Jr., once said: "I saw my mind and heart as flowers. All feelings, passions, sufferings revealed themselves as wonders, yet I remain grounded in my body. There is no enlightenment outside of my own mind and the cells of my body. Life is miraculous, even in its suffering. Without suffering life would not be possible."[2]

What would our lives be like if we honored and explored our darker aspects as much as we hold onto and cultivate our lighter ones? What would happen if we realized that we all move between the pleasant and the unpleasant throughout our journey? Let me answer that. We would be integrated human beings. Feelings would come and go, dancing through us like clouds dancing across the sky. We would have no need to get caught up in fear or anger, no need to hold onto happiness. We would then move into the deep peace that lies behind the dance of opposites, the peace that is our true nature.

The second thing we need to understand is that it is safe to meet our feelings. One of the core reasons we run away from our painful feelings is that we are terrified that they will completely engulf us if we get too close to them. We are also afraid that if we allow them a voice, they will never, ever shut up. Not having been trained to pay attention to our feelings in a respectful and honoring manner, when the rejected ones burble to the surface, we meet them with hatred and fear.

In this rejection, our feelings are just like the snakes Grace Wiley worked with from chapter 5. If someone enters their territory with hatred and fear in her heart, they will attack. So of course we have become terrified of our feelings, for when we attack them, they respond in kind. But just as Grace did with the snakes, we can learn to gentle our feelings with our undivided attention. When we can meet a feeling without running away, it loses its power, and we take our power back.

Using the Four Questions to Explore Our Feelings

Now that we know that it is okay to experience a full range of feelings and that it is safe to meet them all, let us look at the feelings we will meet on our journey back to ourselves. Four basic feelings ask for our undivided attention:

1. *Anger.* This feeling comes from not getting what we want. It can show up as irritation, frustration, hatred, jealousy, rage, criticism, self-judgment, annoyance, resentment, or antagonism, causing us to strike out at life.

2. *Fear.* This feeling is about getting what we don't want. It can show up as free-floating anxiety, unease, panic, alarm, trepidation, apprehension, dread, or terror, causing us to pull back from life.

3. *Despair.* This feeling comes from our sense of nothing ever working out. It can show up as unfulfilled longing, hopelessness, helplessness, sadness, despondency, grief, or sorrow, causing us to give up on life.

4. *Happiness.* This feeling comes from getting what we think we want. It can show up as expansion, fulfillment, excitement, and even thrills. But keep in mind that sometimes these feelings can be too much, moving us into feeling overwhelmed, guilty, and vulnerable. They can even take us into the fear of losing the happiness. Any of these reactions can spin us out of control, causing us to contract again.

To come into a healing relationship with these feelings, we need to get to know them. This is not about collapsing into them; it is about meeting them, giving them the nonjudgmental attention they need to heal. As we explored earlier, being lost in a feeling is the same as saying, "I am so afraid." Meeting a feeling is saying, "Ahh, this is fear." Now let us explore how we can bring the four questions into the world of our feelings.

In This Moment, What Am I Experiencing?

As we cultivate the ability to be present with our experience, we open the door for our feelings to reveal themselves to us. We begin by asking the question, "In this moment, what am I experiencing?" just as we did in the last chapter with our sensations. This question grounds us in our bodies, taking us out of the whirling mind that is always trying to understand, fix, or run away. As we fine-tune our ability to bring our attention into our bodies, it becomes safe enough for our feelings to make themselves known.

Begin by focusing on the strongest sensation in your body and explore it with your attention. As the light of your attention begins to work its magic, the feeling generating this strong sensation can reveal itself. You may notice emotions welling up within you, or you may recognize a familiar story in your head. Whatever begins to happen under the light of your attention, describe it to yourself. Let go of the story around this feeling and be fully present with the experience. What does it feel like? If it is fear, is it a feeling of overall anxiety, or is it a dark knot of dread? If it is anger, is it fiery and explosive, or just a slow burn? Remember, there is no need to judge, analyze, or deny what is there. Be willing, at least for a moment or two, simply to be present. As you let go of your story around this feeling — for example, it is good, it is bad, it will be here forever, I am bad for feeling this, it will take me over — you can then give it the attention it needs to heal.

You can also describe exactly what is happening by writing it down or speaking to another person, as we explored in chapter 7. As you are doing this, you are developing a part of yourself that is not lost in the feeling. Naming the truth of your experience, either by writing it down or by speaking it out loud, allows you to *relate to* it rather than being lost in it. This is a major step in healing, for what your feelings need more than anything is your ability to be present for them. *The feelings that fuel your compulsion have been waiting your whole life for you to respond to them rather than to react.*

A skillful way to deepen your response is to say to whatever feeling is present, "I see you. I'm here." As you say this, you have taken another step into relating to the feeling rather than being lost in it. The power of this statement is that it lets the feeling know it is being recognized and that it is not alone.

Let us take the experience of a lump in your throat. As you make contact with this tension, telling it that you are here for it, waves of sadness may show up, maybe even tears. Along with this may come the feeling of being very alone or maybe of being a failure. Don't second-guess what happens. Whatever needs to show up will. Stay present for the feeling by saying, "I see you, _____. I'm here." Fill in the blank with whatever feeling you have discovered.

Although it may seem that just shining the light of our compassionate attention on our feelings is too simple, the effects of doing this are profound. What happens to you when somebody simply bears witness to your experience without any desire to judge or fix you? It is deeply healing. As you feel recognized and heard, something inside you begins to open. This also holds true for your feelings. When you step out of the normal mode of denying and dominating and instead meet the truth of your experience in a nonjudgmental way, things begin to move and transform.

When you get this close to what you are experiencing, you may find yourself getting lost in the feeling. When you notice that you are struggling again, come back to bearing witness. If things are confusing, ask the first question again: "Now, what am I experiencing?" Remember, these are boxed-up parts of you that need your undivided attention. They don't need you to get lost in them, losing your perspective along the way. Rather, they need you to *see* them and offer them nonjudgmental acceptance.

We also need to understand that *we are not paying attention to our sensations and feelings to make them go away.* That is just more of the same old, same old that we have been doing forever: "I don't like it, and I will try to get rid of it." There is only one problem with that. It doesn't work. Instead what we are doing here is making it safe enough *for the feeling to let go.* There will be times, just as there were when you explored your sensations, when you do not have a clue about what is going on. That's okay. Just the willingness to be curious for a few moments is powerful in and of itself. If, after you have asked, "In this moment, what am I experiencing?" nothing becomes clear, you can ask the open-ended version of the question, "What is asking to be seen?" If nothing reveals itself after a few moments, let the question work its magic underneath your conscious awareness.

Be patient. We are retraining our knee-jerk reaction to run away. In the beginning this happens much like a Polaroid picture developing, with your attention as the developer. Don't rush it — this is a gradual process. If nothing happens, it is okay. Your willingness to turn toward your experience makes it safe enough for your feelings to reveal themselves when they are ready.

I want to share a story from my life that demonstrates how powerful it is to notice and then bring your nonjudgmental attention to the sensations in your body, allowing the feelings that are fueling them to reveal themselves. In my early years of awakening, and usually when I was very tired, I would feel great frustration if somebody took my turn at a four-way stop or if they cut in line in front of me. I would fume and fuss self-righteously. Of course this did nothing for my peace of mind. Then one day I finally became curious. What is so upsetting to me?

The next time I noticed this feeling of righteous frustration was while I was standing in line at the grocery store. I was feeling very rushed, and the grocery store clerk was flirting with the customer before me and taking her sweet time about it. There was a knot in my stomach that was growing tighter and tighter. Before I had learned how to be curious, I simply would have reached over to the display by the checkout stand, picked up a couple of candy bars, and added them to my grocery cart (all the while unmercifully judging the grocery store clerk and maybe even giving her a few ugly looks as I left).

This time I became curious instead. Since I had lots of time (it didn't look like this was going to be a short flirting session), I closed my eyes and took a few deep breaths. I then made contact with the knot in my stomach. As I acknowledged this knot and allowed my attention to rest there, I heard a very young voice inside of me say, "It's not fair! I'm important too." In a flash, I realized that this was the part of me that had grown up in relationship to an older, very dominant sister. I always had to be second in everything. This part of me was vigilant about the "big sister of life" who would shove me out of line or take my place again.

I knew this was one of those boxed-up feelings, because my mind's immediate response was shame. "Such a childish response," it said. But I was present enough to remember that this was just a very young part of me and the rage that it carried was really about all the *second bests* that happened when I was little. Until that day at the grocery store — except for moments when it would flare up and make a mess of my life — this feeling had been closed off inside me since I was very young.

I said to this part of me, "I see you; I'm here." Immediately the rage lifted, and the candy bars didn't look at all interesting. I was even able to be present with the grocery store clerk and in fact thanked her (silently!) for flirting long enough for me to meet this part of myself.

The wonderful thing about being present with feelings is that initially you don't have to stay with them very long if you aren't ready to. Just a moment or two in the beginning is enough to start opening the doors to your healing. As we have explored throughout this book, the healing power of attention is transforming.

At times this can feel scary, for it is the opposite of how we have been trained — which was to resist, run away, and deny. And even though resistance may give us a temporary break from the deep unease inside us, the unexplored feelings in our lives don't go away. They sit there inside us like a low-banked fire waiting for the tiniest bit of wind to flare them up again into a conflagration of compulsions. Relating to them, not resisting them, is the path to freedom.

For This Moment, Can I Let This Be Here?

In the beginning we will discover many feelings that won't dissolve under the light of our attention. That is what these next three questions are about. They are the processing questions, and they bring spaciousness, compassion, and wisdom to our experience.

The question, "For this moment, can I let this be here?" is all about cultivating spaciousness, a necessary component in our healing of feelings that fuel our compulsions. These feelings were buried deep inside us at a time when we had no other way to deal with them. And without our even noticing, they unconsciously drive our actions, causing us to live from the "*I am not* knots" in our minds, bodies, and hearts. Because these feelings are so young, they often won't lose their power over us until they are given permission to exist! Honoring them as they are is the key. It gives our feelings the acceptance they need to heal.

The feelings that most need the spaciousness of acceptance are usually the ones we have hidden deep within the basement of our bodies, the ones we are absolutely ashamed to let anybody know that we have. And we aren't just afraid of what other people may think about our full range of feelings; we are also afraid of letting *ourselves* see the truth of our experience. Part of us feels that if we let on to ourselves about these unacceptable feelings, we would die of the shame.

A wonderfully freeing truth can help you immensely in healing all the boxed-up feelings inside you: *You are not original in the depth and breadth of crazy, vengeful, sad, whining, terrified, petty, overwhelmed, prideful, larcenous, and all-around unpleasant thoughts and feelings that you experience.* In just being alive you have, at one time or another, felt the full range of feelings that are possible for a human being, from pure victimhood to murderous rage. If you doubt that you have ever felt mad enough to want to really hurt someone, watch a two-year-old when somebody thwarts him or her! Then remember that at one time you were a child too.

So the truth is that we're all nutty as fruitcakes. But that is okay. Can you feel the deep breath that comes from accepting the full range of feelings within you? This is not permission to act on them. Rather, it is permission to acknowledge that they are there. The truth is that you are far less likely to act on these thoughts and feelings when you can accept their existence.

Offering this acceptance to your feelings is one of the most powerfully transformative things you can do. When you give something space to *be*, you allow it to move and change. Giving something space is so powerful that if a feeling is not responding to your attention, it is probably because a part of you still doesn't want it to be there. Big surprise! The reason you boxed up your feelings in the first place was that you hated and feared them. So why wouldn't there be a part of you now that resists acknowledging them?

To truly make space for a feeling (remembering that the ones that most need this spaciousness are the ones you have most deeply hated and feared), you need to understand that every feeling you have is as valid as the Earth turning on its axis or as winter unfolding into spring. It doesn't matter if it is illogical or inconvenient. It doesn't even matter if it is irrational. The deep ones usually seem that way if we try to understand them in relationship to what is going on now rather than what was happening when we boxed them up.

You also need to understand that giving a feeling space to be isn't about allowing it to take over your life. *It is about allowing the feeling to be there without your becoming lost in it.* It is the difference between feeling angry or saying, "Ahh, anger." To increase spaciousness, we can use the powerful statement, "It is okay that you're here." This is different from saying, "I see you. I'm here," which is about letting the feeling know not only that you recognize it but also that you are here for it.

The statement "It is okay that you are here" is about giving the feeling permission to *be*. We are conditioned to *do* something with our feelings to get them to change. That is often what we try to do with our loved ones — we feel we have to fix them, change them, let them know how they need to be different. But in healthy relationships, both people have learned to listen to their partners, accepting them for exactly who they are. In fact, the quickest way to effect change in a relationship is to allow the other person to be exactly where he or she is. And the same is true for our feelings.

I would like to share another story that reveals the power of letting our feelings know that their presence in our lives is okay. It is one of the most powerful healings I have witnessed. A brother of a friend of mine who had been diagnosed with a brain tumor called me. He was concerned about my friend, who had retreated to his bed for two months, hardly eating or drinking anything and not wanting to live. After that phone call I flew back East to work with him.

I stayed with the family for five days, and every day my friend and I would spend hours exploring all the feelings coming up inside him. He had had a very intense spiritual life, but he focused on making contact with a higher self and leaving all this mundane earthly stuff behind. This belief had never brought him the peace he longed for; it also had not given him any skills for working with the great initiatory process called illness.

For the first two days, we worked with his deep sadness over possibly leaving his family, the despair of feeling like he had never fulfilled his life purpose, his deep self-judgment, and the fear of the unknown. As we explored all these, he was able to see each of them from a different perspective, and he felt quite relieved. Rather than fighting where he was in his life, he began to open to it and was experiencing quite a bit of peace.

But he would get tripped up on his anger, most of which he projected onto his wife. No matter how spacious he became through our work, at times when he came into her presence the light would go out of his eyes and his whole body would tense up in resistance. The first few times it happened, he didn't have the willingness to be curious about this feeling. While he had been able to explore all his other feelings, when it came to anger he became lost in making her wrong rather than meeting his own feelings.

I knew this feeling needed to vent and be heard. As I listened, I waited for an opening, and when it came, through the question, "In this moment, what am I experiencing?" I asked him to turn his attention within and report what was there. He could feel a tight knot in his belly, and as his attention settled there he began to feel the anger. Through the power of the second question, he was able to let go of the story about his anger, the story that kept him lost in the idea it was all his wife's fault. As he stayed with his own experience he explored the knot in his belly, and began to recognize the rage of a lifetime. I kept repeating to him that it was okay for it to be here and that it had been trying to get his attention his whole life. He began saying to the rage, "It is okay that you're here," and for the first time in his adult life, he was actually present with it. His heart began to open, and with tears rolling down his cheeks, he clearly saw that this feeling had been closed up inside him at a very early age, only to control his whole life.

What came to him then was an image of himself as a young boy, right before he had to hide his rage deep within. He could feel his aliveness, his exuberance, and his joy. Then he watched as the fear he had of his rage (especially in relationship to a stepbrother who was six months older than he) caused him to close down so tightly that he lost sight of his joy. As we talked together later that day, he said he now realized that his whole life had been lived in relationship to this rage. He could look at almost all the decisions he had made and see that many of them came from the need to keep this rage at bay. But now death was looming on the horizon, and it was getting harder to run away.

Two days later, right before I left, his anger was triggered again so deeply that his whole body was shaking. He asked me to come to his room, and he lay down on the bed so that he could clearly feel what was going on. After our work of the past five days, he could now easily turn his attention to his body, find the knot of energy that was his rage, and give it his undivided attention. He was able to stay with this feeling longer than ever, exploring it in depth. Much to his amazement, the waves of rage began to turn into waves of love. He was lying on his back, and tears of joy were streaming down his temples. Every once in a while he would say, "I always thought I had to do something with it."

This is a man who had tried every therapy he could think of. Now he was simply giving his feelings his undivided, nonjudgmental attention, allowing them space to be. In this spaciousness, the energy encased in those feelings was transformed back into joy. My friend had awakened to the power of simply telling himself the truth of what he was experiencing, giving it the space to be, and then letting it know that it was okay that it was here.

He told me that this was the first time in his adult life that he had really wanted to live. He also said he had more energy than he had had for a long time. Of course! All the energy he had spent keeping the rage boxed up was now available for the joy of living. A week later I called him to check in. He told me that the process was continuing and that he was able to meet the feelings that were arising with curiosity and compassion. His family also reported to me that he was eating and drinking now and was spending more time with them. Giving our feelings permission to be truly is transformational.

In This Moment, Can I Touch This with Compassion?

Along with permission to be, our feelings also respond deeply to an infusion of love. Most of our feelings have their roots in deep fear. The word *afraid* comes from the root word *frai*, which means "beloved, precious, at peace." When we add the prefix *a*, which means "away from," the word *afraid* means "being away from the state of feeling beloved, precious, and at peace." To give our feelings an infusion of love is to give ourselves the experience of being beloved, precious, and at peace. We can also become free. For if we can love whatever comes into our lives, what we are struggling with loses its power over us.

Every one of our feelings simply wants to be recognized and loved. But some of them are so young and so scared that they are easily spooked. These are the ones that need a deep and nurturing love to become free, and it takes a number of "love infusions" before they truly understand that you won't reject them again. These are the feelings that will teach you that you can't let go of anything you haven't embraced.

Buddhist teacher and author Jack Kornfield tells a poignant story about a woman who, after spending a lifetime struggling with a degenerative disease that caused pain and weakness, finally discovered the power of infusing whatever she was experiencing with understanding and mercy. As her heart began to open, she saw how much resistance and hatred she had sent into her pain. She decided that if the work given to her was to sit with a body in pain, she would bring to it all the tenderness and mercy she could. As she embraced her pain, she discovered a peace she had never known.

It is a healing moment in our lives when we recognize that all these feelings we have been running from our whole life deeply long to be recognized and understood. To meet them with our hearts can dramatically lessen their power over us. One of the most powerful things we can say to these feelings when we finally recognize them is, "It's okay. I understand." That statement says directly to the feeling, "I hear you!" and is a powerful way to generate the experience of compassion. An example from my own life reveals the power of these four words.

My sister was visiting from Los Angeles at the same time that my son was visiting. And even though I love both of them with all my heart, there were three people living in a small house. We were also visiting a lot of different family members, and I still had to work.

Needless to say, it was a very full time. I also was building a meditation pond in my yard, a project that started out very small and quickly mushroomed into a huge undertaking. After a whole week of struggling with trying to build a water filter, at the end of a very busy day and right after I discovered that my roof was leaking, I discovered that I had been building the wrong filter and that I needed to start over from scratch. Not only did I have to go out and buy all new supplies while throwing the old ones away, but I also had to call my neighbor and ask for more help, which brought up an old fear of being a bother.

On hanging up the phone I froze, feeling overwhelmed. Even though I have experienced it thousands of times in my life, I couldn't say exactly what I was feeling. All I knew was that I was hurting and wanted to run from my life. This was always when I would eat and eat and eat. Instead I went into my room, sat down, and closed my eyes. Taking a few deep breaths I began to ask the question, "In this moment, what am I experiencing?" Letting my attention settle in my body, I began to feel tightness in my chest that felt like a vise around my breath. As I spoke the truth of what I was experiencing, it let go a little and it became easier to breathe.

As my attention became sharper, what I noticed was a dropping sensation right below my chest, the same feeling I would have had if I were on a scary roller-coaster ride. As I stayed there, the feeling of being overwhelmed became clearer. I heard the words that went along with it: "This is too much. I'll never figure my way out of this. I need a break and I can't get one, so everything is going to get worse." I knew it was important to allow this feeling to *be,* for if I fought it, I knew it would only get worse. When I asked if I could let it be here, all I got was resistance. I took a few deep breaths and then asked, *"How* I can I let this be here?" Quickly it became clear that what this feeling needed was the space to be. I began to say, "It's okay that you are here."

As this feeling felt heard and accepted, the despair that was underneath it welled up. It was so deep it needed more than just my recognition of it. It needed to be touched by my heart. As I asked how I could bring compassion to this, I saw how young this feeling was and how it wanted to know that it wasn't alone. So many, many times in my life when it had risen to the surface I had run away from it as fast as I could, abandoning myself when I most needed myself. I began to rock back and forth, saying at the same time, "It's okay. I understand," cultivating compassion, the essence of the third question. I said it over and over, and it brought up very healing tears.

I wasn't saying these words to an idea or a memory. I was saying them to the actual feeling in my body, a feeling that had been frozen since my childhood and had been triggered by everything that had been happening that day. Slowly, as I stayed there giving this feeling my nonjudgmental attention, much like the sun coming out from behind the clouds, I came back to myself. I felt such joy for being able to be that present with feelings that I had run away from so many times in my life. I then went back into the living room to be with my sister and my son. My son, having experienced me in this overwhelmed place many times when he was growing up, said later that he had never seen me move through that feeling so quickly.

You can amplify compassion by holding a hand out, palm up, and allowing it to fill with all the love you can imagine. Then you bring the hand to the area in your body where you are experiencing contraction and cradle it in tenderness. I have also been known to sit down, put both of my arms around myself, and rock back and forth, back and forth, all the while saying to myself, "It's okay. I understand, and I'm here now. It's okay." I have brought even the most terrified parts of myself out of the corners of the basement through this technique. Sometimes I even needed to put a heating pad on my body and enfold myself in a quilt before the feelings felt safe enough to reveal themselves.

It's Okay

To amplify the healing power of the first three questions, we have been exploring three statements — "I see you, I'm here"; "It's okay that you are here"; "It's okay, I understand." These statements deepen our meeting of our feelings and can be boiled down to just two words: *it's okay.* These words move us back into our center where we know, from the core of our being, that no matter what is happening in our lives, *it is all okay.* Everything that happens to us is a part of our journey back to ourselves. And at the truest level, *it is all for us.* It *is* all okay. This doesn't mean that it is necessarily pleasant. We will have all sorts of challenging, scary, and very unpleasant experiences on our journey back to ourselves. But these words allude to the truth that a greater process is taking place. Even the deepest of challenges open us back up to a deep and trust-filled relationship with ourselves and with life.

If you have moments when feelings are moving through you with such power that it is difficult to remember anything we have explored together, just take one deep breath and say, "It's okay." If you feel completely calm, you can still use these words. They can become a talisman, reminding you that this moment is exactly as it needs to be and that everything is all right. The power of adding these two words into your life is enormous. I have given talks based on just this phrase, and people have come up to me afterward and even contacted me weeks, months, and years later. They want to share with me how deeply these two words have changed their lives.

Ultimately, *it's okay* opens the door to our hearts. When cultivating an openhearted relationship with our feelings, it is important to remember that this is a process. We have closed our hearts to ourselves for many years, and some of our feelings are very, very locked up and hidden far away. That is okay. Each time we can be present for our feelings and touch them with our hearts, even for a moment or two, they melt a little more, coming out of the dark and into the light.

Right Now, What Do I Truly Need?

After you have worked with one or with all of the first three questions, it is helpful to ask the fourth question in order to listen for what you need to do, say, or be that is for your highest good. As we have explored throughout this book, you have an inner radar that knows exactly what to do in any given situation. It knows when to say yes and when to say no. It knows when to stop and when to go. It knows when to lie on the couch with a good book. It knows how to eat, exercise, work, and play in ways that bring balance to your whole being.

As you use the fourth question, "Right now, what do I *truly* need?" in your treasure hunt, you reawaken this inner radar. This reawakening allows you to trust your own gut knowing, which can identify better than anybody else how to respond to the feelings that you are now recognizing. Also, every day you are a different person. You have lived a little longer, growing more deeply into yourself. Thus, your needs during every wave of compulsion can be different. There are no pat answers on the journey to healing. This is why questions are so important and specifically why the questions, "Right now, what do I *truly* need?" and its open-ended version, "What is the way through this?" can be of such help.

At the beginning, you may not hear a thing. Ask anyway, for every time you do, you energize your inner radar. The more we ask it, the clearer we get. It is like the silt in a glass of water. As it begins to fall to the bottom, the water becomes clearer.

As we open the space of wisdom through this question, choices that serve our highest good become clear to us. We make skillful choices depending on two different qualities within us: what I call our "Ha quality" and our "Ah quality." The Ha quality (remember the wood-chopping exercise from the last chapter?) comes from the firm and benevolent *no* that we all have within us, and I call these choices wise choices. The Ah quality comes from an open and tender heart, and I call these kind choices. You can get the flavor of these choices by saying these two words out loud. *Ha* is short and clipped. *Ahhhhh* is long and soft.

To understand how to use these two seemingly opposite choices, we need to remember that working with the feelings that fuel our compulsions is like working with a two-year-old. A skillful parent knows that a child acts out at times because she is scared, and all she needs is a few moments of pure attention and some deep-hearted understanding. This comes from our Ah quality, which we have explored throughout this book. Most of the feelings that we will meet on our journey back to ourselves are in desperate need of the heart inherent in this kind of choice.

A skillful parent also knows that there are times when the child needs boundaries and some very clear directions. This is about tapping into our Ha quality in order to make wise choices. It may be just saying to the child, "That's enough." Or he may need a timeout in his room. This is true for our feelings too. There does come a time in our journey when we can say to a feeling or to our compulsion, "No. We are not going there."

This is a new kind of no. Formerly our no was *against* what we were experiencing. We either hated or feared what was going on and wanted to get away from it as quickly as possible. This empowered no is not against anything; rather, it is a wise and benevolent no that is *for* the good of the whole. Just like with parents of young children, when they can see what is going on without reacting to it, their no has authority, and the child recognizes this. In working with these two types of choices, always go to the Ah choice first. Pull in all we have explored on keeping your heart open, both in this chapter and in chapter 8. Then if you feel that it is appropriate to put some limits on your feelings, do so by calling on your empowered no.

I had to work for quite a while to truly open my heart to the deep feelings that fueled my compulsions before I could utter a skillful no. When I said no before I had touched these feelings with my heart, it only made it worse. *As I learned to open my heart to the full range of feelings moving through me, my feelings began to trust that I truly saw them and understood.* Then, and only then, did they begin to trust my no. And it was only when I finally discovered my empowered no that I could take my power back from the thoughts and feelings that had run my life.

So the question, "Right now, what do I *truly* need?" taps us into the empowerment of wise and kind choices. You can directly ask this question of whatever feeling you are experiencing by changing it slightly and saying, "What do *you* need right now?" The more connected to your feelings you become, the more you recognize how desperately they need us to be there for them. They respond deeply to our willingness to ask them what they need and our willingness to listen for a response.

But sometimes you may not be able to listen — you may not even be interested in listening. This will happen many times on this journey back to yourself. In these types of situations you can ask the fourth question in an open-ended way: "What is the way through this?" Remember, this is the default question. This is the one to ask when you aren't sure what to do. It works even if you are still lost in doubt and confusion.

Listen as deeply as you can. If nothing comes and you feel in need of some direction, ask yourself what a friend or loved one would do if he or she were in this same situation. You can also go back to the Lost Child

Meditation from chapter 8 to see exactly what it is that you need. If it is still not clear, imagine asking the advice of the person you admire most in the world.

It is also helpful to imagine how doing the exact opposite of what you are doing right now would look. If you are feeling quite closed, go outside and take a walk. If you are moving at a frantic pace, take a break. If you are judgmental, cultivate your heart. Remember, this fourth question taps you into a wisdom that is much greater than anything your mind can come up with on its own. Keep asking, and know that the questions are working for you.

As we learned while working with sensations, what we truly need at every point in our lives is a deep connection with life, right here, right now. So after we have met our feelings and given them whatever they need — even if all we can do is recognize for just a moment that they are present — one of the wisest choices we can make is to place our attention on the immediacy of life.

The more we do this, the more we will understand two important things. The first is that we do have a choice about where we are going to place our attention. The second is that all the reactions in our minds, bodies, and hearts are just a small fraction of what is going on in this moment of our lives. You don't have to stay caught up in the never-ending story in your head and all the reactions it breeds in your body and emotions. Instead, you can open the field of your attention and rediscover life, with all the joy and wonder that is available right here, right now. You are alive! Your heart is beating. Your breath is rising and falling. Your body is glowing with the gift of life. In some profound way, all the struggles of our lives — especially our compulsions — are part of a process that is bringing us back into this full connection with the only moment that matters: *now.*

As we become more present in this process, sometimes we will be able to let go of all our struggles and open to the newness of life, here and now. Other times we will need to consciously cultivate opening, lifting our attention from the narrowness of our struggle and placing it onto something else. We can walk, dance, bake, sing, bike, sit quietly in the garden, read a book, rent a movie, or call a friend. Gratitude also opens us again, as does generosity, especially the generous gesture of being there for another person. Remember: our old patterns have a momentum that has been growing for days, months, even years. But when we see how our reactions cut us off from the pure joy of being alive, it becomes easier to let them go and to bring our attention back to the fullness of life right now.

It is best to practice this opening after you have worked with at least one of the first three questions. To try to open ourselves again without at least a few moments of responding to our contraction just fuels the cycle of reaction. But as we meet our experience, even for a moment or two, we begin to discover that nothing in our old story of struggle can ensnare our attention, drawing us into a spiral of reaction. Not only that, no matter how many challenges we may be experiencing, we can easily return to the fullness of life, right here, right now.

There is a statement that can help define the difference between being caught in our story and being fully present for life: "This is it!" It reminds us that this moment is a gift. These three words say that everything that *has happened* in our lives belongs to the already lived. And everything that is *going to happen* isn't yet here. They remind us that life is happening right here, right now, and this is the only moment that matters. One day we won't have any more moments, so let us be fully present for the ones we are given.

The words "This is it" reconnect us with the living adventure of life. This adventure isn't always pleasant, but it is much more painful and exhausting to stay closed than it is to open. As the Moody Blues song says, "It is easier to stay than to turn around and run!" When my mind says, "Why would I want to be present for a headache, or a noisy room, or a whining child?" I remind it that resisting only makes it worse. I also remind it that resistance cuts us off from everything we truly long for. So I invite you to pause for a moment, let go of all your ideas about life, and be fully present with wherever you are. See the space you are sitting in. Hear the sounds all around you and within you. Feel the pulsating aliveness of your body. Be here. This is the living moment of your life. Then from this place of responding to life rather than reacting, listen for the kinds of choices that will bring balance and harmony into your life.

Enhancing the Questions with Our Breath

Deep breathing is a powerful tool in this process of returning to ourselves, for it can keep us spacious in so many ways. Just as breathing techniques can help a woman while she is giving birth, the same is true for us as we are giving birth to ourselves. This is why we spent so much time on breathing in chapter 9 and touched on it again in the last chapter. The most basic thing you can do with your breath is to keep breathing as you explore your immediate experience. Because the process of turning toward what we are experiencing and exploring it with curiosity and compassion is so new to most of us, we often unconsciously hold our breath. To add even one deep breath can be very freeing.

You can use two breathing techniques to bring more space to your feelings. The first is an amplification of the Balloon Breath we did earlier. As you take in a deep breath, gently expanding your area of contraction from the inside out, imagine that you are infusing this area with deep tenderness and care. Then on the out-breath, imagine all this contraction melting like ice does in the warm summer sun.

The other breath technique is my version of an ancient Buddhist practice called Tonglen. Through compassion, this technique not only can help you meet the most contracted feelings within you, it can also transform the world. Let us experience it together.

Exercise

Once you have read through the exercise, begin by closing your eyes and allowing your attention to rest on the rhythm of your breath. As you settle in, let your breath deepen, bringing a sense of spaciousness inside you. You can add pauses at the end of the out-breath and the in-breath to intensify your experience if you wish.

Now bring your attention to the center of your chest and remember the warmth and the radiance that we breathed into ourselves in the Ball of Love meditation we did in chapter 8. Breathe in and out of your heart area for a few minutes and let this ball of light expand and glow with warmth and love.

Now bring your attention to any physical or emotional pain that you may be experiencing in your body. Feel as specifically as you can the sensations that are appearing as this pain. If you can't find any pain, imagine a pain you have had in the past. Then just like a vacuum cleaner, on the in-breath pull whatever you are focusing on straight into the healing radiance of your heart. See it dissolve just like ice dissolves in the warmth of the sun. If you like to visualize, you can imagine it as dark smoke being pulled into your heart and then being transformed into pure light.

On the out-breath, send waves of radiant warmth from your heart into the area that is in pain. Stay with this breath for a while, breathing your pain into your heart and then sending clear, radiant light back on the out-breath. If you want to, you can also send an opposite quality into your pain. If you are experiencing fear, send courage on the wave of your out-breath. If it is anger, send compassion. If it is confusion, send clarity. If it is despair, send the knowledge that you are not alone.

When this feels complete, bring into your mind's eye another person on the Earth who is experiencing the same pain that you are. It could be a child, a friend, a loved one, or even a stranger. Realize that, just like you, they are suffering and long to live from the healing of the heart. Again, just like a vacuum cleaner, breathe their pain straight into your heart. Let it be touched by the transforming energy of this radiant light. On the out-breath imagine waves of warm, loving, compassionate energy flowing from your heart to them. See them being transformed right before your eyes. When you are done, open your eyes.

When There Is No Release

We need to remember that it takes time to heal the core feelings that run our compulsions. We have hidden them deep and run from them hard for many years, often for many decades. But sometimes there is not enough space in our consciousness to see or enough mercy in our hearts to meet the feelings coursing through us. When nothing else seems to be working, we can give ourselves two gifts:

Asking for Help

No words can express how central to our healing the ability to ask for help is. In fact, it could be said that all the challenges in our lives are given to us so that we'll be confounded enough to ask for help from the wisdom at the heart of life. When you finally understand that help has always been waiting for your request, and when you see how much easier your life becomes, you will wonder how you ever lived without asking for help in this way.

One of the simplest and most powerful ways to ask for help is to use the open-ended questions: What is asking to be seen? How can I give this space to be? How can I bring compassion to this? What is the way through this? It would be useful to reread the section on open-ended questions in chapter 12. This will help you to remember that you are living a very specific process, and whatever is happening in your life is a part of your journey back to yourself. It will also remind you that the Intelligence that gave you life, including all of your challenges, is always close at hand.

Moving Your Energy

As we explored in the last chapter, getting our bodies moving can be very helpful. It is now reported that for milder cases of depression, a ten-minute walk is more effective than antidepressants!

Moving our bodies is not the only way to move energy. It can also be done by allowing someone to hold you and to simply be there without words. If no one is around, you can hold yourself. One of my favorite gifts to myself when I am feeling vulnerable and overwhelmed is to make a nest of my bed, putting on multiple layers of comforters, and burrowing down deep inside.

We can also use exaggeration to get our energy moving. This can be a lot of fun. If I am mad, I love to yell and scream and rant and rave in my car. I work on getting the yells to come from deep within my body, and, boy, does that feel great. If I am feeling overly responsible, I love to go to my neighborhood park and swing. If I am judging myself, I will sometimes go to the mirror and say, "Oh, boy, you really screwed up, didn't you?" with a little twinkle in my eye. I then give myself a list of supreme screwups about the most ridiculous things — "You drank out of the wrong side of your teacup this morning! You even put on your left shoe before your right. And besides that, you didn't hang up your towel perfectly!" I think you get the gist. It is all done in the name of maintaining perspective, for being truly alive is about screwing up part of the time — and some days even a little more often than that!

Even though a good deal of the time moving energy is very freeing, when we are contracted we all carry an inclination to stay closed. From the prison of contraction, opening looks very, very scary. So each of us has our own brand of resistance to moving when we freeze again. I used to be afraid of going outside when I felt particularly frozen. It was just too much space! As I began to honor my fear of going outside when I was contracted, I became willing to push its boundaries a bit, which I found very freeing. I now can go outside even when I am sad or afraid, and I find that rather than contracting, I become more spacious.

Listen to yourself to find out whether moving your energy is appropriate. Your inner radar will tell you what needs to be done. Every time it will be different. Be willing to push the envelope of your resistance just a bit, and watch what happens. If what you do causes you to resist even more, be gentle. It is okay to let yourself stay frozen. Simply in recognizing that you are too scared to move, you have moved your energy by touching yourself with your heart.

In this chapter we have explored ways to bring the light of our compassionate attention to all the feelings that fuel our compulsions. Many of them will dissolve under the light of our pure attention. And the ones that don't will usually dissolve under the light of understanding and mercy. For feelings, just like people, become healthy and balanced in the face of nonjudgmental attention. At times you will only be able to feel the sensations in your body. That's okay. The more you turn your attention toward yourself and notice what is going on, the more the feelings will reveal themselves. Over time you will be able to go directly to the feeling and meet it with your compassionate attention, and it is this quality of attention that will dissolve the feeling. It is also important not to push the river. There will be times to go toward a feeling, and there will be times to move away from it. Many of the feelings that are asking for our attention are very, very young, and it is essential to respect their timing.

Know also that at the beginning, a moment or two of meeting will probably transform a surface feeling but probably not the deeper ones that are fueling your compulsion. *But every time you meet a feeling, even if it is for only a brief time, it loses a little more of its power over you.* Over time you will be able to meet the most hidden feelings inside you and transform them through the light of your compassionate attention. This is what they need to heal. It is not in changing, getting rid of, or denying our experience that we will know the peace we long for. It comes from being in direct relationship with it. As Robert Frost once wrote, "The only way out is through."

Core Ideas

- To come into a healing relationship with our feelings, we need to get to know them. This is not about collapsing into them but about meeting them, giving them the nonjudgmental attention they need to heal.

- It is safe to meet our feelings.

- Because these feelings are so young, they often won't lose their power over us until they are given permission to exist.

- Your willingness to turn toward your experience creates enough safety for your feelings to reveal themselves.

- When we can meet a feeling without running away, it loses its power, and we take our power back.

- The three statements — "I see you, I'm here"; "It's okay you are here"; and "It's okay, I understand" — dramatically heal your feelings. Your feelings have been waiting for a long time to hear these words.

- Everything that happens to us is a part of our journey back to ourselves. And at the truest level, *it is all for us.* It *is* all okay.

- The statement "This is it!" helps define the difference between being caught in our story and being fully present for life. It reminds us that each moment is a gift.

- When you finally understand that help has always been waiting for your request, and when you see how much easier your life becomes, you will wonder how you ever lived without asking for help from the wisdom at the heart of life.

Chapter 15

TREASURE HUNTING WITH

Compulsions

I n this final chapter about treasure hunting we will draw on everything we have explored together so far and bring the transformative
power of the four questions to our compulsions. First let us do a
brief review of our new way of looking at and healing our compulsions:

1. *Compulsions are not the enemy.* If we treat our compulsions as
    the enemy, we get caught in an endless war, fighting forces that
    are much stronger than our attempts to control them. Rather,
    compulsions are a part of a survival system that we needed
    before we learned how to be present with ourselves. We are not
    compulsive because we are weak-willed ninnies, helpless in the
    face of powerful urges that are trying to destroy us. These forces
    that confound and confuse us are here to awaken us — to open
    us back into a deep and abiding relationship with ourselves and
    with life.

2. *Compulsions come straight from life's longing for us to reconnect with who we truly are.* We are all given the exact set of circumstances in our lives that we need to come out of the attic of the mind, back into the house of our *being*. Compulsions are one of the greatest teachers in this shift from contraction to connection. Because they are more powerful than any of our attempts to control them, they push, prod, and cajole us into responding rather than reacting. They refuse to leave us until they teach us to be curious about what we are experiencing and compassionate with everything we discover.

3. *Lasting healing takes place when we can be present for whatever we are experiencing in the moment.* Whenever we are compulsive, instead of turning away we need to turn toward our experience. Rather than always managing our experience, we need to learn how to engage with it, shining the light of our compassionate attention on it. In other words, the essence of healing is the understanding that ultimately we don't need to fix or change, hate or fear our compulsions. What we need to do is be present with them and touch them with our compassionate hearts.

4. *Our compulsions bring close to the surface everything inside us that is asking for our compassionate attention.* When we meet what we are experiencing with curiosity and understanding, our boxed-up feelings lose their power to fuel our compulsions and to control our lives. Then the energy that was bound up in our old patterns is released back into the free-flowing aliveness that we truly are.

5. *As we reconnect with ourselves, instead of being trapped in our familiar mode of reaction and struggle, we experience an ever-deepening joy and an abiding trust in ourselves and in life.* Eventually we come to know and live again from the entire house of our being, connected to the wellspring of deep knowing within. This is the greatest gift compulsion has to bring to us — this ability to

reunite us with our wellspring, which is connected to the Creative Intelligence at the heart of life. This great and wondrous Intelligence that beats our heart and breathes our breath then becomes our partner in this marvelous adventure called life.

Using the Four Questions to Heal Our Compulsions

To see what our compulsions are trying to teach us, we need to become more interested in what is happening inside us than we are in getting lost in our compulsions or in trying to control them. The four questions hold the keys to doing this. They retrain our reactive minds so we can see and be with *what is.* They also tap into the deep knowing within that will guide us every step of the way on this journey back to ourselves. Instead of exploring each question, as we did in the last two chapters, here we will discover how to bring the four questions to the different phases of compulsion, focusing both on our sensations and our feelings.

Most compulsions come in waves. There are three phases to a wave: the beginning, the middle, and the end. Here we will begin with the end of the wave, for that is the easiest place to learn the art of engagement. It is a treasure trove of information that can allow us to take our power back from our compulsion. We will then explore the middle of the wave, where we are fully engulfed by our compulsion, usually losing clarity, connection, and mercy. This is the place where we can see what it is that is fueling the wave of compulsion and bring it the healing of compassion. And finally, we will explore the wave just as it begins. It is here that we can relearn how to make kind and skillful choices that empower us to our core.

After the Wave Has Passed Through: Breaking the Spell

Because we have been so unconscious about our compulsions, the tendency to fall into them and pull the covers over our head is very strong. So asking ourselves to be curious about what is going on when the wave is building or after we are fully lost in it can be difficult at the beginning.

It is when the wave has passed through and the cravings have subsided sufficiently that we can peek our heads out from under the covers and see what is really happening.

After the wave has passed through, we can do two things to minimize the power of our compulsion. The first is to be truthful with ourselves about the price we pay for being compulsive, and the second is to see through the heavy states of mind that try to grab hold of us at this time.

Recognizing the Price We Pay

After a wave of compulsion has passed through, we usually stay in reaction, losing the opportunity to recognize the price we pay for taking care of ourselves in this way. We all know that compulsions wreak havoc in our lives, but we usually are not willing to truly feel what we are experiencing. Instead we stay stuck in our heads, using this information to try to get ourselves under control. We often pull ourselves up by the bootstraps and declare that *now* we will be in charge. "Never again will I allow my compulsion to get the best of me," we say.

For a time we feel a sense of power as we start another diet, dump the pills down the toilet, throw away all the alcohol, cancel our Internet provider, promise to end our workday at five o'clock, or cut up the credit cards. But there comes a day, if we haven't yet met the feelings that are fueling our compulsions, when the urge to fall into our compulsion resurfaces more strongly than any resolve we may have mustered.

To take a breath and ask the question, "In this moment, what am I experiencing?" in the aftermath of our compulsion allows us to see, and *finally to truly feel* with great clarity, the heartache that comes in its wake. This is true whether it is the rages of a food hangover, the anxiety that dogs us when we can't ever get to the end of our to-do list, the pervasive smell of cigarettes, the price our family and social life pay for our being a workaholic, or the despair we feel when our credit card is denied: *the short-lived satisfaction of our compulsions simply isn't worth it.* Even if we do find a small amount of peace, we can finally see that it doesn't last. We can then open to the possibility that there are easier, kinder, and more lasting ways to take care of ourselves, ways that enhance our lives rather than leaving us struggling and disempowered.

To clearly *feel* the price you pay, as soon as you surface out of the wave, acknowledging that you've been lost in your compulsion again, ask, "In this moment, what am I experiencing?" Focus on the sensations in your body, for that is usually where you will most clearly see the price you pay for your compulsions. This question turns your attention into a flashlight, highlighting what is happening. Describe whatever you discover there: headache, tightness in your throat, acid stomach, butterflies, overall tiredness, difficulty breathing. Be as specific as possible. You may find it helpful to review chapter 13, where we explored tuning into our bodies through noticing our sensations. Remember that the power of naming something is awesome. *In that moment you are relating to it rather than being lost in it.* If feelings — anxiety, sadness, dread, irritation — reveal themselves, name them too. Every moment that you can be present for the habitual patterns of sensations and feelings in your body that come on the heels of your compulsion, you lessen the power of your compulsion. If it is hard to see or be present for your feelings, review chapter 14 to further develop your capacity for curiosity and compassion.

If overeating is your compulsion, notice what it feels like when you overeat. Does your heart pound? Is there a bad taste in your mouth? Is your stomach upset? What happens to your emotions? Do you hate being in your body? Are you lost in despair? Be as curious and as real as you can with the least amount of self-judgment you can muster. Then ask yourself, "Is this my heart's desire for my life?" This question invites you to step out of judgment or despair and really look at what is happening right now and see if this is how you want to live. Be careful with this question. If it fuels more judgment and despair, then let it go. There will come a time that this question will bring you deep clarity about what your heart truly desires for you.

If you drink, explore what it feels like to wake up with a hangover. How does your body feel? How does it change your emotions? In what ways does it make the next day more difficult? A powerful way to break the spell of overdrinking is to ask a friend or loved one to videotape you when you have had too much to drink. Then ask yourself, "Is this my heart's desire for my life?" If your compulsion is shopping, notice that the wonderful feelings don't last very long — both the warm, cozy feeling of being in the store and the thrill of your new purchases. Especially notice what it feels like when you recognize how much money you have spent. Also be truthful about the subterfuge that goes along with overspending — hiding your activities from yourself and your loved ones. How does this hiding and lying make you feel? And is this your heart's desire for your life?

You can be truthful about any compulsion. For example, ask yourself what it's like to wake up with a stranger in your bed. How do you feel about the smell of cigarettes on your clothes, the constriction in your lungs, or being ostracized by nonsmokers? What happens when, after seeming to be on top of your "to-do" list, you feel the sense of despair that comes from not getting everything done?

To amplify this process of acknowledging the truth of your experience, you can write down what you discover, either in an Awareness Diary, as we discussed in chapter 7, or in free-flowing writing. You are not writing to change anything. Rather, you are doing this to discover that compulsions never bring you what they promise — in fact, they do the opposite.

It can also be helpful to make a list of everything you discover after a wave of compulsion has moved through. Write down, point by point, your sensations and feelings. When your compulsions come knocking on the door, you can take out your list, which will remind you that compulsions don't give you what they promise, and this can help with making wise and kind choices. It can also be helpful to share this list with a friend or counselor — someone who won't judge you if you fall into your compulsion again and who will not try to use this information to make you stop being compulsive. He is simply there to bear witness to your truth. When somebody listens to you, you can begin to listen to yourself. This brings you out of the fog of denial about the havoc your compulsion will wreak.

To pay attention to the price we pay for being compulsive brings the first ray of light onto our pathway back to ourselves. Paying just a little bit of attention begins to break the vicious circle of going to our compulsions for help, being devastated by them, and promising never to indulge again, only to get seduced once more and then falling into the self-hatred and despair that fuel the next cycle of compulsion. When compulsions cast their spell again, promising that if we follow them they will give us all the comfort and peace we long for, we can remind ourselves of the price we will pay for believing them.

Seeing through the Heavy States

When a wave of compulsion has moved through, we often get lost in the core feelings that fuel our compulsions: fear, self-judgment, and despair. And as we get lost in them, they make us vulnerable to another wave of compulsion. To break the spell cast by these feelings, let us take an in-depth look at them, for if we can see how they operate, we can become free of them.

Fear. Can you recollect the fear that comes after a wave of compulsion? It usually makes itself known when the numbing aspect of compulsion wears off and you realize, "Oh no. It came again!" You experience both the fear that you will never be free of your compulsion and the fear of the consequences you will now have to live through. Fear can contract you so much that all you want to do is crawl back into your compulsion. If you overeat, you may experience the fear of gaining weight. If nobody knows about your compulsive activities, then the fear of being found out will come rushing in. If your compulsion affects your health, the fear of what will happen to your body can be paralyzing.

To run from our fear only makes it worse. It is only by *meeting our fear* that we take our power back from it so it won't fuel another wave of compulsion. Meeting our fears, though often terrifying in itself, can bring true freedom. As Eleanor Roosevelt once said, "You gain strength, courage and confidence by every experience in which you really stop to look fear in the face."[1]

If you are spinning in confusion after the wave has moved through, you are most likely feeling fear on some level. Asking the question, "In this moment, what am I experiencing?" can focus your jumbled mind. Then if you find fear — perhaps the free-floating anxiety that restricts your chest, the ball of dread in your belly, or the band of tightness in your head that signals trepidation — explore it with the laser beam of your attention, naming to yourself whatever you discover.

Stay with it as long as you can, *relating to it rather than being lost in it.* You can also work with the next two questions so that you can give this feeling the space and the mercy it needs to be healed. If it works for you, talk to your feeling. This is a very young part of you that needs somebody to acknowledge it, just as children need somebody to acknowledge their fear of the dark. The more present you are to it, the more it will dissolve, leaving spaciousness and clarity in its wake. If you can't be with the fear, be with the fear of being with the fear. It does take courage to meet our fears, but as Mrs. Roosevelt reminds us, standing with fear brings healing.

If you find yourself very angry, this is usually because you are afraid in some deep part of yourself, afraid you won't get what you need. The anger is trying to protect as it distracts you from your fear. If you resist your anger, it either becomes very explosive or it turns inward into corrosive shame. To open to anger is very freeing. Learning how to feel it without being afraid of it or using it for attack, either against ourselves or somebody else, can be a very alive and pleasurable experience. As our anger is freed up, we can then work with the fear that always lurks underneath it.

Self-judgment. The fascinating thing about anger is that it is usually a secondary feeling, happening in response to a deeper feeling. One of these deeper feelings is self-judgment, which is just anger turned within. It is so easy to judge ourselves for being compulsive. We have been trained from a young age that being compulsive is evidence of our weakness and our willfulness. And so we judge ourselves, not seeing that this judgment helps to fuel our compulsions.

The most dramatic story I have ever heard about the power of judgment to fuel our compulsions and the power of mercy to heal them came from a woman I was counseling a few years ago who was a chronic overeater. She took a huge step in her healing when she was able to transform her relationship with her mother, who was in the later stages of diabetes. Her mother's legs were going to have to be amputated. And even though her health was this fragile, she still smoked.

Her mother's smoking brought up judgment in my client that bordered on fury. She felt that her mother should have been smart enough to give up smoking years ago. Because she didn't, my client felt that her mother was to blame for everything that was happening in her body. This fury not only put a wedge between the two of them that was causing great heartache, but it was also keeping my client caught in a struggling mind, fueling her compulsions without her even being aware of it. Part of my work with her was to help her to see that this searing judgment of her mother's behavior was exactly how she related to her own compulsions.

Eventually she realized that her mother had done the best she could with the level of knowledge she had, and rather than anger, she began to feel compassion. Their relationship became dramatically better, so much so that she finally told her mother how mad she had been and how she now understood. When she did this, her mother began to cry. She told her daughter that she was that mad at herself too, feeling that she was a total failure for not being able to stop smoking. She also shared how tormented she had been by this self-judgment. No wonder she needed to keep numbing herself out!

This was an important moment for my client. She finally saw what we had been talking about — that what you try to control only controls you, keeping you caught in a never-ending circle of disempowerment. She was also able to see how important it was to meet compulsions with compassion and mercy. As she met her mother with mercy, she learned how to do this for herself, and her urge to be compulsive dramatically lessened. And when the mother received compassion rather than judgment for her inability to stop smoking, she was able to stop.

The period after a wave of compulsion has moved through can be one of the hardest times to become merciful with ourselves, but it is also one of the most powerful. Because self-judgment can be so seductive, we can use the second and third questions to break its spell: "For this moment, can I let this be here?" or "For this moment, can I touch this with compassion?" You can even get more specific with this question by asking, "Can I meet myself with understanding and mercy?" The energy of these questions is all about spaciousness and compassion, circumventing our knee-jerk reaction to meeting our experience with judgment and shame. Remember, your compulsions are the way your psyche figured out how to take care of you when you were disconnected from your own truth and wisdom.

If your heart is closed tighter than a drum, you can ask the open-ended question, "How can I give this space to be?" and "How can I bring compassion to this?" These questions are asking our deep knowing to help us to meet ourselves in understanding and mercy. Feel the relief over the fact that you don't have to figure out how to do this. You can also review the skills in chapter 8. The Lost Child Meditation, the Ball of Love Meditation, and the Voice of Kindness can each open your heart again so that self-hatred cannot get a foothold inside you, fueling another wave of compulsion.

Despair. After a wave of compulsion passes through, the other core feeling that sometimes engulfs us is despair. This despair tells us, "This is hopeless. I will be caught forever." Although despair may be harder to let go of than self-judgment, it is still an untruth. Nothing lasts — neither our difficult experiences nor our joyful ones. They are all a part of a river of experience that is heading back to its source. And the difficult ones are not present because we have screwed up or because the higher power in charge of it all has fallen asleep on the job. The challenges in our lives are openings rather than closings. They are doorways into the healing that we long for. As Albert Einstein once said, "In the middle of difficulty lies opportunity."

To dismantle despair, you need to realize that you are a growing and continuously changing process. As you unfold, you are being shaped by powers much greater than you. You are like those breathtakingly beautiful trees by an ocean that are sculpted by the great forces of nature. If you watch a limb being torn off in a wild storm, you may feel despair that the tree is being marred. But over time you can see that this pruning by the forces of life gives the tree its unique beauty. You too are being shaped by powerful forces, and one day you will recognize your perfection exactly as you are.

Despair also tells us, "It is bigger than I am. I will never be able to stop this." Both these statements are true. Compulsion is bigger than any of your attempts to control it. Thank God! And you are not the one who can heal it. There really is something bigger than you in charge, and this presence stays with you every step of the way.

There will be times after a wave of compulsion has moved through when you are not interested in discovering the price you pay for being compulsive; times when your mind and heart are too jumbled to work with fear, self-judgment, and despair; and times when it is all so confusing that you don't have a clue about what is going on. This is the time to use the fourth question: "Right now, what do I *truly* need?" This question points you in the direction of listening to the wisest part of yourself that knows how to bring balance back into your life.

If your mind is too foggy to see the most healing thing to do, or if it is too resistant even to listen, you can ask the fourth question in an open-ended way: "What is the way through this?" This default question is extremely helpful in working with whatever shows up inside us after a wave of compulsion has moved through. For just a moment or two you can let go of reaction and sincerely ask for help.

Again, you don't have to get an answer or even know who or what you are asking this question of. This question is like a ray of sunshine breaking through the stormy clouds on a dark winter day. It points to the presence of something bigger than you that is waiting for your request for help. The sun may shine for only a moment, but that one moment reminds you that even though the cloud cover is thick, the *sun* of support is always with you. So let the question set things in motion, even if you don't feel a thing.

During the Wave: Meeting Your Feelings

As you break the spell of compulsion by paying attention after a wave has moved through, allowing yourself — without judgment — to fully feel the effects of following your compulsion again, one day you will find yourself in the middle of a wave, and you will suddenly be aware of what you are doing. The story I recounted in chapter 5 about sitting with ice cream in my lap and a whole row of cookies lined up along the back of the couch was the first time this happened to me. It was like waking up out of a dream and, without judgment, becoming very curious about what I was doing.

This is such a powerful time in a wave of compulsion. Here you are running away as fast as you can, while running toward an imaginary cessation of your pain. With the information you gained by paying attention after the wave has moved through — that it never brings what it promises and instead it makes you feel worse — you can stop running away and turn to meet yourself instead. We can give ourselves two things at this time — the curiosity to see what is going on and the healing of compassion.

Passionate Curiosity

The first step in meeting your feelings is to see what is going on. This isn't just *thinking about* what is going on. This is actually *experiencing it.* Turning toward yourself in this way is how you can begin to heal. With the light of your attention you can meet the feelings that are fueling your mad dash to numb out.

Remember the Wicked Witch of the West in the film version of *The Wizard of Oz?* She had such power over everybody's life, until Dorothy discovered that the witch dissolved when water was thrown on her. That is the same power our attention has when we can bring it to whatever we are experiencing in the middle of a wave of compulsion. We can learn how to use our attention to dissolve whatever is there just like water dissolved the witch.

Imagine yourself in the middle of a wave of compulsion — maybe you are eating a large pizza on your own and rather than feeling better you are feeling more despair. Or maybe you are lost in your to-do list, absolutely furious at the line at the post office because it isn't going to let you get everything done. Or it could be that you are lost in a pornographic website that isn't bringing you the high you were looking for.

Rather than being lost in the experience, you find yourself becoming fascinated by what is happening, and it is this curiosity that breaks the ever-tightening grip of compulsion. In the beginning you will probably only be able to be present for a moment or two, since the urge to run away is deeply programmed. But every time you turn toward your experience, you lessen the power of your compulsion.

It is extremely helpful at this time to get out pen and paper and just start writing. This is less formal than writing in your Awareness Diary or making a list of your experiences. This is writing down everything you notice without concern for how neat it is. It is a little like being in the middle of a tornado and noticing different objects as they fly by. Write down the sensations, thoughts, and feelings you discover as they appear and disappear inside you. After the wave has moved through, you will have a document that describes the inner working of your mind, body, and heart when you are caught in a wave of compulsion. This information is absolutely invaluable. It is so powerful to do this that it doesn't matter if all you have to write on is a napkin. Capture what is going on by writing it down, and you will be able to see the depth of the pain that fuels your compulsion — the depth of pain that needs your compassionate attention. Eventually you will be able to be present for whatever you are experiencing in the middle of a wave of compulsion, which will powerfully diminish its impact. If you are keeping an Awareness Diary, you can also go back later and lift out of this free-flowing writing some of the core patterns you can now see and then note them in your Awareness Diary.

If nothing comes clear when you ask the question, "In this moment, what am I experiencing?" you can ask it in an open-ended way: "What is asking to be seen?" For whenever we are compulsive, something needs our attention. As you ask this question, pause for a moment, and if a sensation or feeling reveals itself, pay attention to it. If it doesn't, let it go, knowing that the question will work its magic. Over time all the feelings that fuel your compulsion will reveal themselves, not to be fixed or analyzed or understood, but simply and powerfully to be seen and transformed in the light of your compassionate attention.

A close cousin to the question, "What is asking to be seen?" is, "What am I resisting?" By now we know that whenever we are in the reaction of being compulsive, there is something we don't want to see. By asking to see what we are resisting, the mind becomes curious rather than reactive, and chances are greater that the part we have been resisting will reveal itself. If it doesn't, let the question go, and it will signal life that you are learning how to listen.

Meeting our feelings through these questions reforges a bond of trust. We need to understand that healing our compulsions is much like healing a broken relationship. Neither person trusts the other. Likewise, you don't trust your compulsion because it has caused you so much heartache. And it doesn't trust you, because the only relationship you have had with it has been one of domination and annihilation, never listening. These questions are all *about* listening and will eventually help you not to be so afraid to experience what you are experiencing.

The most basic thing to remember is that whenever you find yourself in the middle of a compulsive wave, ask a question. If you dive right back into the wave again, that's okay. You didn't learn how to walk overnight, and you won't learn how to respond to your compulsion overnight either. At the beginning this one little step may not seem to make much of a difference, but moments such as these have a power and a momentum of their own. They begin to open a door back to you. Once that door is open just a crack, you will feel the relief of being present with yourself — even if you are upset, angry, overwhelmed, afraid, or sad.

The Healing of Compassion

The second step to healing the deep and hidden feelings that fuel a wave of compulsion is to meet them with understanding and mercy. Whatever you discover in the middle of a wave — even if it is the unwillingness to discover anything — will respond to the question, "For this moment, can I let this be here?" This question adds spaciousness and nonjudgmental awareness to the process. You can then go to the third question, "For this moment, can I touch this with compassion?" to access the healing of your heart. If you are too stirred up even to contemplate touching your experience with your heart, you can go to the open-ended question, "How can I bring compassion to this?"

Relearning how to be merciful with the feelings that fuel our compulsion breaks the self-judgment that keeps the cycle going. A feeling may be irrational and very scary, but it loses its power when we can *see* it and then *be* with it, even if it is just for a moment or two. Yes, these are powerful forces, but they are no more powerful than our ability to *respond* to them. The only reason they seem like such monsters is that we have resisted them. Now that we are listening to them, we will greatly reduce their power to engulf us.

The statements we explored in the last chapter can also help immensely in giving our feelings the understanding and mercy they need. Saying "I see you. I'm here." lets your feelings know that you are willing to be with them. Because these feelings can so easily either retreat back under our awareness or flare up and engulf us, the statement "It is okay you are here" opens the lines of communication between you and the feeling. And the statement "It's okay, I understand" can melt even the most angry and terrified feeling inside you. These words can be wonderfully soothing to our feelings, and they can serve as a doorstop, preventing our heart from slamming all the way shut again. These statements are about honoring whatever you are experiencing. Remember, you are not trying to make your experience go away. Rather, you are giving it the space it needs to let go on its own. It may take a while before your feelings feel safe enough to let go as you support them with your full attention. As you do this, you will discover that right behind the feeling is a wide-open space where everything is okay.

This is also the time to cultivate mercy for yourself for being compulsive. Remember, you are not compulsive because you are some weak-willed ninny or because you are defective or broken. Your compulsion is a deeply ingrained survival system that was created because the journey of your life had taken you away from a nourishing and wise connection with yourself. And if you don't judge yourself for being compulsive, choosing compassion instead, your compulsion can show you what needs to be healed.

If nothing is clear, or if you have a compulsion — such as taking drugs or drinking — that directly affects your ability to pay attention while you are compulsive, this is the time to use the fourth open-ended question. Asking, "What is the way through this?" taps you into the wisdom of life and can be very healing in the middle of a wave. Even just a moment of surfacing out of your compulsion and asking this question is a step down the path of your healing.

As the Wave Begins to Build: Empowered Choice

Most of us either are not aware that we are falling into a wave of compulsion until we are completely lost in it or we don't want to acknowledge what is happening. But as we become curious, respecting and listening to our compulsions when they show up, we become attuned to their rhythms. It is then possible to wake up and be present for a wave just as it is beginning. This is when we have the greatest possibility of making choices that are for our highest good. For *where there is awareness, there is choice, and where there is choice, there is freedom.*

There are four ways we can work with our compulsions at the beginning of a wave.

Saying No

When we have gotten to know our compulsions well and have met enough of our feelings with our heart, we have earned the right to say no to the urge to be compulsive when it arises. After all we've explored about how detrimental it is to dominate our compulsions, this may seem confusing at first. This confusion will clear up when you understand that this is a different "no" than most of us have experienced in the past. This empowered no, which we explored in the last chapter, is not about trying to control ourselves, creating resistance in the process. Rather, an empowered no is about discipline, which comes from the Latin word *discere,* meaning "to learn, get to know." Discipline here means learning how to be in relationship with ourselves in a skillful way. It is not about being against a behavior; it is about being *for* kind and skillful choices.

The old type of no comes from feeling hatred and fear toward our compulsions, and the hope that if we can dominate them, they will go away and leave us alone. The controlling mind uses it to try to make us behave. And as we have all discovered, this doesn't work in the long run. The empowered no comes from the very center of our being. "We don't need to go there," it says. It is very clean, ringing like a clear bell throughout our being.

We have to earn the right to an empowered no. Because we tried to dominate our experience using our old type of no, we empowered a very stubborn and rebellious part of ourselves. We say, "I am not going to be compulsive!" and it says, "Oh, yes we are!" That is why so many times we have felt a deep determination never to be compulsive again, only to have the urge flare up and roar through us like a wildfire.

This rebellious one is ultimately a very healthy part of us. It says, "I won't let go until you begin to listen." Every time we listen to ourselves rather than running away, we not only untangle the web of compulsions, but we also gain the respect of this rebellious part of us. When we begin to listen, this rebellious part — whose only option in the past was to numb out through compulsion — begins to see that we are maturing. It recognizes that we are learning how to be present for ourselves and to make choices that are for the good of the whole. It can then begin to respect our empowered no.

And believe me, even though this rebellious part can be truly unbearable at times, opposing our highest intentions, when we discover our empowered no, it is actually glad to have somebody else on board.

It is like an abandoned child who has had to be completely in charge of its own life. Finally an adult has assumed responsibility. The child, after some fussing and fighting, feels great relief.

There may be times, even after living and practicing our empowered no, when we temporarily lose sight of it again. All that means is that something inside of us needs to be met so that we can clear enough space for an empowered no to emerge. In many instances, with the help of the four questions we can free things up enough for this to happen.

An experience I had on September 11, 2001, highlights what we are talking about here. When I turned on the television that morning and learned about the terrorist attack on the World Trade Center in New York City, I stood there in stunned disbelief and grief. Almost immediately the phone began to ring. Rather than being present for my own experience, I became present for other people, which at that time was appropriate. I went on to counsel people individually and then led a group.

After the last person left, I immediately felt the urge to eat and eat and eat. For the first time in ages this feeling was so strong that the idea of going to the grocery store was dangerously seductive. I immediately asked for help by asking my favorite version of the fourth question, "What do I need to do that is for my highest good?" Out of the fog of reaction came the knowing that the only reason I wanted to fall into my compulsion was that something burbling within me needed my attention.

From an empowered place I was able to say to myself, "No, we aren't going to the store." The rebellious part of me said, "Don't mess with me. We're going." Even though I was on the fence, I was able to remind myself that eating lots of chocolate would only make everything more painful in the long run.

Remembering that the wisest thing to do was to become curious about what was going on inside me, I sat in the chair on my front porch. I then asked, "In this moment, what am I experiencing?" What was most evident was the overwhelming urge to eat. Understanding that it was trying to numb something inside me, I then asked, "What am I resisting?" Immediately I could feel the fingerlings of grief that I had ignored earlier in the day. "Can I let this be so I can be fully present with it?" was my next question. This question opened me up, allowing me to honor my grief. As it welled up within me, I cried and cried for the Earth, for all the human beings who had died, and for the people who had lost friends and loved ones on this tragic day. I even cried for the terrorists, for they had to be deeply wounded to plan and celebrate such an act.

Those tears were so cleansing, opening a vast space of compassion and mercy within me. From this clear and present place the wave of compulsion met the shore of my heart and simply evaporated. I was then able to be truly present with all the people I counseled for the rest of the day.

Because compulsion won't let go until it teaches us how to see and be with what we are experiencing, it retrains us to use our minds as we did when we were young — to make contact with life as it is right now. This contact is about getting out of the stories in our heads and instead tasting what we taste, feeling what we feel, and seeing what we see. In other words, *it is about experiencing what we are experiencing.* And this is what, in the deepest parts of ourselves, we are really longing for whenever we are compulsive.

That is what happened for me that day on my porch. After I opened to my grief, I raised my eyes and saw the autumn leaves beginning to turn gold. I heard the music of the waterfall in my pond, and I watched the play of the squirrels in my yard. I was fully *here.* I realized with an even deeper commitment that this was my gift to life, especially to the many people who had lost their lives. They died because of human beings who were lost in their own reactive stories. In these moments, when I have moved beyond my own struggles and reconnected with life, right here, right now, I have become a part of the healing of our troubled planet.

If I could free myself from the struggling mind, then so too could others. As more and more people do this, eventually humanity will wake up enough to reconnect with the spectacular gift that is life and recognize how precious it is. The more we wake up to life, the more our own struggles, rather than being something to struggle with, become a wake-up call. When we find ourselves contracting in any way — tightening our bodies, holding our breath, wanting what is not here, not wanting *what is,* feeling the urge to be compulsive — all become a signal that we have gotten stuck again in the attic of our mind and that we have a choice about whether we will stay there. By simply recognizing what is going on and then by remembering that we don't have to limit ourselves to this old story, we can bring our attention back into the fullness of life and the fullness of who we truly are, right here, right now. The joy of coming home to this moment is a million times greater than any fleeting happiness that being compulsive can bring.

Giving Options

If we can feel a clear no, and yet we still feel a pull to follow our compulsion, this is the time to look at some skillful options. Let us imagine that 75 percent of you feels the empowered no, but the rest of you wants to get lost in your compulsion. When we are this close to stepping away from our old behavior, this is the time to use the information you have gathered by paying attention after a wave of compulsion has passed through, and you can remind yourself that being compulsive doesn't make you feel better. In fact, it will probably make you feel worse. It is important not to use force at this critical moment. Instead, ask the question, "Right now, what do I *truly* need?" Again, this is listening for what you *need,* not what you want. Asking for clarity about your most valid needs opens a doorway to your deeper knowing so you can listen for a way to take care of yourself that brings balance rather than upset.

Remember, whenever you are compulsive, you are searching for the temporary peace and connection that your compulsion brings you. How can you get that peace and that connection in a skillful way? That is what the question, "Right now, what do I *truly* need?" is all about.

Most of the time when you are this close to not following your compulsion, the wisest option is to place your attention elsewhere by doing something else. By doing this you learn that you have a choice about what to focus on. You also learn that there is much more going on in life than just your struggles. You can place your attention elsewhere through physical movement, writing, speaking your truth, singing, dancing, washing windows, and even showing gratitude and generosity.

A powerful time of learning how to give options came for me after the joyous but overwhelming day of my daughter's wedding when the old urge to eat came back. It was like a cornered animal at that point, and I knew I needed to be very gentle. I said, "Yes, you can eat all you want, but I remind you that tomorrow you will feel quite rotten." I was far enough along in cultivating an understanding and respectful relationship with my compulsion that it was able to hear me. The next time I looked at all the food I wanted to eat, it didn't have the power over me that it had had just a few moments ago.

I then asked, "Right now, what do I *truly* need?" The first option I thought of was what I call deep comfort. What I needed was a quilt, an open heart, and the willingness to take care of myself in a way that is kinder than eating everything in the fridge. I said to my compulsion, "Let's go snuggle on the couch." Much to my joy, it let go of its grip, and I was able to choose that option.

Negotiating

Sometimes, as I feel a wave of compulsion encroaching and I offer myself a different option, I will hear some internal grumbling. "I don't want that," says the rebellious one inside me. "I want my compulsion." The rebellious part of you truly believes that being compulsive will make you feel better! It is no accident that it sounds like a two-year-old. That is how young our urge to be compulsive can get. And this is where, just as it would with a small child, negotiation works so well.

You can say, "I understand that you are absolutely certain that you need to be compulsive. Rather than a whole chocolate bar, how about having just a bite or two and really savoring it, letting it melt in your mouth?" In my life, because I have cultivated a kind and respectful relationship with my compulsion, it can usually listen to me and be amenable to negotiation. I discovered the power of negotiation in my relationship to exercise. For most of my life, I treated exercise just like I treated my compulsions — I was demanding and dominating. I would either exercise in ways that were really boring, or I would exercise to exhaustion, only to have all of my have-tos, got-tos, and shoulds foster their opposite: I won't!

So for years I didn't exercise. Because this wasn't helping my health and because all my attempts to muscle myself into submission had failed, I began to create a relationship with the rebellious side of me. I realized it wouldn't even consider the smallest of exercise programs because I had been such a demanding and dominating taskmaster. Now I exercise daily, and with great joy. Of course, I started small when listening and negotiating with my rebellion. I also spent a lot of time noticing and reminding myself how good I felt after I exercised.

Slowly my rebellious side let go of its grip in the face of my willingness to work with it. Every once in a while it will try to take over again and rebel against any exercises. If reminding it that exercising will make us feel better doesn't do the trick, I negotiate with it. I say, "Let's only do fifteen minutes on the bike today." And that usually works. But there are still times when it isn't going to listen to any negotiating whatsoever. And those are the times I say, "Okay. Let's not exercise today." The more I negotiate and listen, the more consistent my exercise becomes.

Choosing Your Compulsion

Sometimes an empowered no is nowhere to be found. All we want to do is crawl into our compulsion and get lost. Our attempts at exploring what is going on and offering options or negotiations fall on deaf ears. All is not lost. There is a reason for whatever we are experiencing. It is part of our path back into a deep and abiding relationship with ourselves and with life.

Remember, we are not compulsive because we are losers at the beck and call of urges that are out to get us. We are compulsive because there is something we need to see, to embrace, to heal in order to become conscious human beings. So when a wave does hit, it is for a reason. And when it doesn't dissipate on the shore of your compassionate curiosity and instead looks like it is going to crash right on top of you, one of the most powerful things to do is to *choose your compulsion.* You literally say to yourself, "I choose to be compulsive." Even though this may seem crazy at first glance, I assure you it is one of the quickest ways to reclaim your power.

Why is this so powerful? Remember what it used to be like at the beginning of a wave of compulsion before you learned how to be curious? You wanted your compulsion, but you didn't want it. It was like driving down the road of life with one foot on the accelerator and the other on the brake. Most of the time the compulsion won, because you fueled it through your resistance. From little urges, your compulsions grew into big monsters when you tried to fight them. You shift this dynamic and take your power back when you simply say, "I choose this!"

Choosing his compulsion was the doorway out for a client I worked with a number of years ago. His core compulsion was drinking. As we worked together, his compulsion calmed down through his curiosity and compassion, and he learned to take care of himself in ways that allowed him to make skillful choices even when he was overly busy and stressed. As he expanded his capacity to see and be with himself exactly as he was, he began to feel his empowered no. He wasn't using this *against* his drinking, he was using it *for* his health and the health of his family, and he began experiencing more and more nights when he didn't need to drink. And when his drinking would flare up again, he always learned something new.

During a crisis at work he had a two-week spell when all he wanted to do was drink again. The urge was so strong that it wouldn't respond to any of the skills he had been learning. At first he was freaked out. "Oh, no! It has come back again, and I will never be free of it." When he came to see me, we worked with that fear, and he remembered that *even though the urge to drink was very strong, it was not stronger than his ability to be curious about it.*

We then began to explore the idea of choosing this period of compulsion. I watched his whole being change as he became more and more empowered. He could see that as long as he fought with his drinking, he lost himself in the struggle. As soon as he said, "I choose this," the energy it took to do all that struggling was freed up, and he could again be curious about what inside him wanted to be healed during this period of compulsion.

The next day, while he was absentmindedly raking leaves in his yard, it came to him with utter clarity that being with his family was more important to him than isolating himself through his drinking. This epiphany wasn't something that he was going to try to *do* in his life. Rather, it was a deep knowing within him that felt right and true. Along with it came the ability to say yes to a balanced and healthy life.

When he shared this experience with me, he was a bit perplexed and at the same time thrilled. He said that for the two weeks leading up to this revelation, he had felt that if he didn't follow the urge to drink, he would be unable to live. The urge was that urgent. And yet now, even when it came through that strongly, when he said yes to it, he could then easily say no with a ring of truth that his compulsion absolutely heard. And rather than falling into a black void, he felt more alive. He was amazed at the power both of his new yes and his empowered no, and so was his family.

Keep in mind that choosing your compulsion isn't giving in to it. It is holding the intention to be curious about what is going on. Curiosity that starts at the beginning of a wave of compulsion is wide-open and spacious. It is a fascination about what you can learn as you consciously move through a wave of compulsion.

To enter a wave of compulsion in curiosity is a little bit like going out with someone for more than six months and suddenly discovering that he has a scar on his nose. It is just amazing to you that you have never noticed it before. You didn't notice because you weren't really looking at this person. The same is true with your compulsion. You haven't been taught to pay attention. When you hold the intention to be spacious and curious throughout a wave of compulsion, *there is always something you can learn.* This is also a good time to ask yourself, with as much compassion as you can muster, "Is this my heart's desire for my life?"

Every once in a while, when I am very tired and very busy, I just need to comfort myself through my compulsion. I then yield to it, but I remind it that I will be as present as I possibly can throughout the wave. When I go through it with deep curiosity, I always learn something more about myself and about my healing. Because of this, I go for long periods without even a hint of a compulsive urge. Also, my waves are much smaller than they used to be (a few bites of a food that isn't good for me rather than a whole package), and their duration is much shorter too.

Meeting ourselves before, during, and after a wave of compulsion is not a logical, systematic process. Sometimes you will be able to be present at the beginning, sometimes only in the middle, and sometimes not until after the storm has blown through. Some days will be easy, and some days will be more difficult. At times it can be scary and overwhelming as you turn toward your experience, and sometimes it will bring the greatest joy you have ever known.

Remember, trying to stay in control and manage your feelings through being compulsive (and trying to manage the compulsion itself) is to live in a low-grade fever of reaction and struggle, never discovering the healing that you long for. To meet and transform your experience through the healing light of attention and mercy is to experience the healing and cleansing fire of purification.

Everything we have explored in these chapters about treasure hunting will eventually help you to transform your old patterns back into the field of aliveness that is your birthright. On this path back to yourself, don't dive right into the core of your compulsion. That would be like going to the gym and starting with the one-hundred-pound weights. All you will do is pull your muscles of frustration and despair. Start treasure hunting with the more everyday experiences of your life — asking the questions when it is just an ordinary day and your compulsion is nowhere to be found. This will strengthen your ability to be curious and compassionate and will remind you not to do everything alone. You will then be able to be truly present when you are compulsive.

A dear friend of mine who has been reading the drafts of this book and working with the skills, shared a story that describes what I am talking about. Her eleven-year-old daughter belongs to a circle of friends who have been together for years. At each of her birthday parties, my friend would set up a treasure hunt for the girls. When they were six, the clues were really obvious — such as "go to the stereo in the living room" — and the treasures would be sitting out in the open. As they got older, the treasure hunt became more challenging. Since the girls had been practicing treasure hunting for years, they didn't find this frustrating because their capacity to listen to the clues and be very curious about what they were pointing to was increasing along the way. My friend said that you could watch their developing minds rising to the challenge.

She told me that the process was the same with her. When she began to treasure hunt with her own life, it took her a while to be curious about her compulsions. She had been trained, like all of us, to react and control. She first had to start with little things — her irritation at the length of the stoplight, the slight headache at the end of a busy day. She then cultivated the ability to ask the questions in the middle of her daily challenges. Finally she was able to be truly present for herself when she was compulsive, and wise choices became much easier to make.

As you treasure hunt in your life, understand that there will be times when you will be able to incorporate all four questions in an instant. At other times you may need to explore only one, and for only a moment, before you need to distract yourself. Or you may find yourself spending more than an hour with just one or two of them. Time does not matter. Just the willingness to turn toward yourself in curiosity and to open your heart, just for a moment, takes you another step along the path to your healing.

Don't rush yourself. What we are talking about here is a healing *process*. So let all that we have explored be seeds planted in your consciousness. Don't turn our explorations in this book into *have-tos*. Let the seeds grow in their own time and their own way. You will then become like a new shoot that has grown for a long, long time up through the dark winter soil and has now found the light. Since it is not yet spring, some days will still be very cold, and some days will carry the riotous promise of spring. To allow the new green shoots of your healing to blossom into the fullness of who you really are, don't force things. Your deep inner knowing knows how to allow you to unfold until, in your own time and your own way, you fulfill your promise, giving your true beauty and essence to the world.

Core Ideas

- *Compulsions are not the enemy.* If we treat them as the enemy, we get caught in an endless war, fighting forces that are much stronger than our attempts to control them. Rather, compulsions are a part of a survival system that we needed before we learned how to be present with ourselves.

- To see what our compulsions are trying to teach us, we need to become more interested in what is happening inside us than we are in getting lost in our compulsions or in trying to control them.

- Most compulsions come in waves, which come in three phases: the beginning, the middle, and the end. Within each wave lies a treasure trove of information that can allow us to take our power back from our compulsion.

- We finally realize that compulsions never bring us what they promise — peace and comfort — and that, in fact, they bring the opposite.

- Our compulsions refuse to leave us until they teach us to be curious about what we are experiencing and compassionate with everything we discover.

- When a wave of compulsion has moved through, we often get lost in the core feelings that fuel our compulsions: fear, self-judgment, and despair. If we can see how they operate, we can become free of them.

- Your empowered no is not about being against a behavior; it is about being *for* kind and skillful choices.

- Treasure hunting with the everyday experiences of your life will strengthen your ability to be curious and compassionate and will remind you not to do everything alone. You will then be able to be truly present when you are compulsive.

- Don't rush yourself. What we are talking about here is a healing *process.* So let all that we have explored be seeds planted in your consciousness.

- *Love is.* Let it in.

COMING FULL

Circle

L ike all the heroes in the great myths about finding lost treasures, in this book you have been invited to partake in a mythical journey, a journey back into a deep and abiding relationship with yourself and with life. This process takes time and courage. (Courage, by the way, comes from the French word *coeur,* or "heart".) And as in all the great myths, the rewards far outweigh the rigors and perils of the journey.

Because this book has come into your life, you are already on this journey back to yourself, with your compulsion as your guide. Some days will be easier than others. Some days you will be able to let go of the urge to be compulsive, and some days you won't. Some days you will be able to be merciful, and some days you won't. Some days you will use all that we have explored to try to stop your compulsion, and some days you will use it to be curious. Some days you will be able to live in the questions, and some days you won't be able even to remember them. Some days you will be able to stay present for yourself, and some days you will need to run. Some days you will be able to pause and remember that it is all a part of a wise and benevolent process, and some days you will be filled with doubt and fear.

At times you will feel like you are making lots of progress, only to experience what feels like backsliding. But there is no such thing! The old adage that life is about taking three steps forward and two back is just a perception of the human mind. It is all forward progress, even when it seems like everything is falling apart. Life is a very intentional, highly organized process that offers you exactly what you need to awaken. There will come a time when you will be able to see and to live in the truth that life can be trusted, opened to, and fully lived.

Even though it takes time to unravel the web of compulsion, what we have explored in this book is really the shortcut. If we use the story of the tortoise and the hare as an analogy, we are like the hare, thinking we can dash to the finish line by managing our compulsions. As we fail over and over, we find ourselves back at the starting line again. In the meantime, the tortoise, which is slowly and surely opening the boxed-up parts that fuel compulsions, gets closer and closer to the finish line.

Even though it is gradual, and even though it is difficult at times to be present with your experience, it is well worth it. Know that each moment that you turn toward yourself with curiosity and understanding is another step on the path to freedom. Each time you can open rather than close, even if it is opening to how closed you are, and each time you can respond rather than react and connect rather than contract, is a healing moment.

Without your even noticing it, there will be longer times between the waves of compulsion, and when the waves do come they won't be so overwhelming. You will become more merciful with yourself and others and more trusting about the unfolding of your life. The pendulum of experience will still swing from side to side, but you will be fascinated by it rather than being stuck on it, endlessly swinging from one reaction to the next. And the more fascination you feel, the faster you will respond to a wave of compulsion when it comes.

As you relearn how to open to life, you will forget and remember and forget and remember what we have explored a thousand times. It doesn't matter. It is all a part of the process of awakening. Tens of thousands of people have walked this path before you and have experienced the same remembering and forgetting. And tens of thousands will walk after you, aided by your willingness to return over and over to the life and the challenges you have been given.

Whenever you find yourself despairing, feeling that you have lost your way, just take one deep breath and say, "It's okay." For whether you feel it or not, it is. And if you need a deeper remembering, go out and lie down on the earth. Feel her holding you as you dance through oceans of space and see her breathing through you the river of breath that is life. Then imagine the possibility of having a deep and abiding love affair with yourself and with life. Imagine a life of vibrancy, authenticity, trust, peace, and spontaneity that is a pure joy to experience. It is possible to be this connected, to be this comfortable in your own skin. It is possible to trust yourself and your life so much that you are healed to your core. It is not only possible, it is your birthright.

The wonderful thing about healing and being healed by your compulsion is that it isn't just for you. As you heal, so too does the Earth. The challenges you have been given are challenges we all experience. Your compulsion has been experienced by presidents and by teenagers. That self-hate you get lost in is felt by great opera singers and by children living on the streets of Calcutta. The despair that overtakes you is experienced by people living in abusive relationships and by world leaders trying to make a difference. The fear you know so well is felt by children going to school every morning and by the parents who are seeing them off. You have been given your compulsion and all the fear, self-hate, and despair that come with it to wake up. And as you meet yourself with understanding and mercy, you clear the pathway for every other human being to be healed in this way too.

So be willing to show up. Tuck the words *it's okay* into your heart, and then open to your life. Live in questions so that they become a beacon of light on the path back to you. Be curious. And over and over, pause and *open to your life,* however it is in that moment. Everything you need is right here.

I would like to leave you with two poems I wrote as a part of a Christmas gift to all the people with whom I work. I used the picture of the Earth that was taken from the moon on the Apollo 11 mission and wrote these words on the black velvety space that surrounds the Earth:

We are so much more than we think we are.
Be still. Listen.
Hear the truth of who you really are.

On the back of the picture I wrote:

It is the human heart that will see that we are all in this together, floating on a tiny blue green jewel through vast oceans of space. It is the human heart that will recognize that Love is the ground of being out of which it all arises.

By Love I mean the field of pure potentiality that is the connective tissue of the universe. It not only holds all of Life together; it animates and nourishes everything from the inside out. This includes atoms, molecules, cells, rocks, panda bears, people, planets, and you.

It is Love that will reveal to us how to show up for the path we have been given so that we can become Love waking up to the truth of Love. And it is Love that will give us the courage to be who we truly are.

Appendix

HANDY REFERENCE GUIDE TO SKILLS AND
Techniques

Below I review many of the skills and techniques we have explored together, along with a few new treasures to tuck into your heart. These may look like the smallest of things — almost insignificant — and yet they are powerful beyond words. As the old saying goes, "Great things come in small packages." This is certainly true for each of the gifts we can give to ourselves when we're facing our compulsions. I have put them in alphabetical order rather than trying to list them by priority, since at any given time any one of these skills may be better suited for you than another.

Ask for Help

·The belief that we are alone is at the heart of all human suffering, and it shows up dramatically with our compulsions. Our attempts to control them only enhance our sense of isolation and the corresponding belief

305

that only we and we alone can free ourselves from our heartaches. It could be said that one reason our compulsions arise is to bring us up against the belief that we have to figure everything out all by ourselves. They hang on till we get a glimmer of the truth that we truly are not alone.

Asking for help is powerful. Jesus alluded to this power when he said, "Ask, and it shall be given you; seek and ye shall find; knock and it shall be opened unto you. Everyone who asks, receives; and everyone who seeks, finds." One powerful way to ask for help is open-ended questions. Besides the question "What is the way through this?" two of my other favorites are, "What is love's wisdom in this moment?" and "What do I need to say, do, or be that is for my highest good (or the highest good of everybody concerned)?" After years of working with this last question, it all boiled down to just two words: "Show me." Whenever I say this, I am telling the Intelligence at the heart of life, "You have given me this challenge, and I am open to your wisdom and support in moving through it."

Sometimes the answer will come immediately, and sometimes it will take longer, for answers come in the time and manner that are for our highest good. *But be assured that answers will come.* So be willing to ask and keep asking. The help that is always there for us simply awaits the opening of a question.

Be Merciful

One of the core reasons that we have been cultivating the ability to be curious is so that we can be present enough to touch ourselves with our hearts. As Saint-Exupéry's beloved character *The Little Prince* said, "One sees clearly only with the heart. Anything essential is invisible to the eyes."[1] Healing is about meeting ourselves with understanding and mercy, and no matter where we are in a wave of compulsion, what we truly need is mercy. Just saying the word *mercy* over and over can have a very healing effect. This opens a space around whatever we are experiencing. If this word is not enough, reread the end of chapter 8.

Here are some other ideas and techniques that can help in opening your heart again:

- Forgive your compulsion. It has been trying to take care of you.
- Forgive yourself for being compulsive. It is not a defect; it is a doorway.
- Be a self-judgment sleuth. See what your shaming voices are doing rather than believing what they are saying.
- Imagine what you would do for a child who is experiencing what you are experiencing. Then give whatever you discover to yourself.
- Imagine what someone who really loves you would say or do for you, and then say or do this for yourself.
- Know that your perfection includes your imperfections!
- You are enough!
- Open your heart to see how closed your heart is.
- Acceptance is magic.
- Accept whatever is happening in your life. It is okay. You are okay.
- You are worthy of love.
- Live in the question, "What is the kind choice here?"
- Live in the question, "How can I bring compassion to myself?"
- Look at yourself in the mirror and wink!
- See all your feelings as little children in need of your understanding and mercy.
- Use the three statements "I see you, I'm here"; "It's okay you are here"; and "It's okay; I understand."
- Breathe tenderness into your pain.
- Rock yourself.
- Bring your hand to your heart.

Breathe

Breath is a magical tool that is available no matter what is happening in your life. When you become connected to the deep and powerful healer of your breath, everything in your life becomes much easier. Breath is all about reconnection. Whenever you are compulsive, you are hungry for connection with yourself and with life. Breath provides this connection through opening what has been closed, calming what has been turbulent, and clearing what has been cloudy.

Take just one deep breath. If you took breaths throughout your day, the chances of your compulsion taking over would become a lot slimmer. And even if it does, breath can keep you open so that you can gather all the treasures that lie hidden in a wave of compulsion. You can also try the Balloon Breath to open up a physical or emotional space that is contracted, the deep natural breath to calm the mind, the Breath of Fire to clear things up, and the "Ha!" Breath to open up emotions.

Live in Questions

Live in questions! Live in questions! Live in questions!

I can't say enough about living in questions. With the check-in questions you learn how to be present for yourself, lifting the clouds of reaction, opening the prison gates of your heart, and listening to something deeper than your reactionary mind. With open-ended questions you tap into support and clarity, no matter what is happening in your life. Remember, you aren't asking questions to figure anything out. The wonderful thing is that you don't have to be curious, trustful, calm, or even clear to ask questions. All you need to do is ask. The questions will work their magic from underneath your everyday awareness. Play with the two sets of questions. Also revisit the list of other questions in chapter 12. If none of these questions calls to you, then use the question, "What are my questions?" And when all else fails, ask the fourth open-ended question over and over: "What is the way through this?" Allow this question to fan the tiny flicker of trust that knows that open-ended questions tap into the wisdom at the heart of life. Following is a quick review of both sets of questions, along with their intents:

The Four Check-in Questions

1. In this moment, what am I experiencing?

2. For this moment, can I let this be here?

3. For this moment, can I touch this with compassion?

4. Right now, what do I *truly* need?

The Four Open-Ended Questions

1. What is asking to be seen?

2. How can I give this space to be?

3. How can I bring compassion to this?

4. What is the way through this?

The Intent of Each Question

1. The intent of the first question is to pull our attention out of the story in our heads so that we can see what is going on right now.

2. The intent of the second question is to help us stop fighting what is going on so we can give it the space to heal.

3. The intent of the third question is to allow us to touch our experience with the healing of our hearts.

4. The intent of the fourth question is to help us listen to the deep knowing within us that is waiting to help us through the opening of a question.

Move

Your essence is a field of free-flowing energy, a field of aliveness and joy. When you are compulsive, you have closed yourself up, contracting into patterns of holding and resisting. Underneath that contraction is the longing to be open again so that you may know and live from the joy that you truly are. Whenever you feel contracted, ask the wisest part of yourself how you can open up again. Breathing is the simplest, but not the only, way. You can sing, dance, walk, swing, skip, clean the house, shake your body, yell at the top of your lungs.

Remember, when you are contracted a part of you wants to stay that way. It truly feels that staying contained is safer. But the truth is that safety comes from opening to the process life is giving you and allowing it to take you where you need to go.

Remember

When we are compulsive, the parts of us that don't know how to trust, to connect, and to love have taken us over. That is why at times it can be so hard to remember what we have explored. We have been trained in contracting and reacting. What we are exploring here is its opposite — opening and responding.

We can do two things to help us remember what we most need to remember when we need to remember it. The first is to go back through this book and write down the ideas and techniques that call to you. If you have underlined passages, use those. If you haven't, open the book randomly, begin to read, and write down on an index card whatever feels right to you. With these notes, you will have a written memory of exactly what will help you back to your center. You can tuck them in your pocket or purse, tape them to your mirror, put them on your refrigerator, or use them as bookmarks.

The other thing you can do to help remember is to write down the four questions and put them in your car, all over the house, and even at work. I have put them in the refrigerator, under my pillow, on the dashboard of my car, on my toothpaste, across from the toilet. You can write all four down, or just one. Whenever you come across them, pause and ask at least one of them. And whatever response you get is exactly what is supposed to be, even if it is resistance to the questions!

Say Good-bye

There does come a time to say good-bye to your compulsion. Though it is part of a survival system that you needed at one time, as you rediscover a deep and abiding relationship with yourself, you will no longer need this old system. When you say good-bye you acknowledge all that your compulsion has given to you and taught you. You are also affirming that you are choosing healthier ways to take care of yourself.

This good-bye may contain some sadness; this is normal, for you are grieving the loss of an old way of finding comfort and connection. One of the ways you can say good-bye is to light a candle every day for a week to honor your compulsion and, as you do this, thank it for all it has taught you. You can write letters to your compulsion and then burn them. You can buy a greeting card that acknowledges the end of a relationship and then send it to your compulsion at your address. There are many ways to say good-bye. If it is time, let your good-bye unfold as it will.

Speak Your Truth

Speaking our truth is what the first question is all about — to experience what we are experiencing. I cannot stress enough how important this is on this journey back to ourselves. Over and over, I listen to people who are struggling and then find themselves struggling with their struggle and sometimes even struggling with the struggle that they are struggling with! (Are you following me here?) What they say over and over is that stopping for a moment, asking, "In this moment, what am I experiencing?" and then speaking the truth of it to themselves cuts through the story about what they are experiencing so they can experience it! Some part of them, even if they are very reactive, knows that acknowledging what is happening is a way out of the maze of struggle.

We can amplify what we discover in two ways. Both bring our experiences out of the shadows inside us into the light of day where we can more clearly see them and then see through them. The first is to write it down. Wherever you are in a wave of compulsion, you can get out a pad of paper, ask yourself, "In this moment, what am I experiencing?" and start writing. Put a pen to paper and let it flow. Nobody is going to look at what you've written. You can burn it right after you are done if you need to. Writing this way is the safety valve on the pressure cooker of your experience. Keep writing what your experience is right now. You can also keep an Awareness Diary, which we explored in chapter 7. The second way to clarify the truth of your experience is to speak it to another person. It can be helpful to set up a contact person in advance — someone whom you trust to listen and not judge, and someone fairly easy to get a hold of. Then, when you discover yourself in a wave of compulsion, call them and speak the truth of what you are experiencing. Remember, they are not listening to help you, to fix you, or to judge you. They are simply listening so that you can listen to yourself.

Take a Refreshing Pause

To break the spell of compulsion, it can be very helpful just to pause for a moment, feel your breath, and become aware that a lot more is going on in your life than just the urge to be compulsive. Life, in all its wonder and beauty, is unfolding within you and around you right now! To pause can also remind you that you are a part of a greater process. There are more stars than there are grains of sand on every beach of the Earth! And all life dances in such synchronicity that we can time the returning of the morning sun to a millisecond. You are a part of a highly intelligent, highly organized unfolding, and the river of your experience, especially your compulsion, is exactly what you need to become a truly conscious human being. And this moment is the only moment in life that truly matters. It is a doorway into everything you have truly longed for and into who you truly are.

Tell Yourself It's Okay

These two little words — *it's okay* — are a core part of lasting healing. When you try to control something, it controls you. When you fight something, it fights back. Saying "It's okay" takes you out of reaction and calms things down. As you let go of struggling with what is going on, you can begin to see more clearly what you need to do that will be for your highest good in any situation.

So tuck these words in your heart and say them in all situations — when you're feeling tired, frustrated, compulsive, overwhelmed, sad, mad, confused, or all the above. For they can take you out of the struggling mind, opening the doorway into the wellspring of wisdom and love that is always with you.

Thank Your Compulsion

It takes the wind right out of our compulsions' sails when we thank them. A compulsion is just like a lumbering beast made up of old patterns, and it thinks it has to take care of you in this way. When you thank it, it becomes putty in your hands, for it deeply responds to appreciation. In fact, it loses its power in the face of gratitude.

Notes

Introduction

1. Mary O'Malley, *Belonging to Life: The Journey of Awakening* (Seattle: Awaken Publications, 2002).

Chapter 3
Recognizing Our Compulsions as Friends

1. Gregory A. Kimble, *Principles of General Psychology* (Hoboken, NJ: Wiley, 1980).

Chapter 5
Moving from Management to Engagement

1. Jelaluddin Rumi, "The Guest House," from Coleman Barks, *The Essential Rumi* (San Francisco: HarperCollins, 1995), 109.
2. J. Allen Boone, *Kinship with All Life* (New York: Harper & Row, 1954), 95.
3. Mary O'Malley, *Belonging to Life: The Journey of Awakening* (Seattle: Awaken Publications, 2002), 174.
4. O'Malley, *Belonging to Life,* 174.

Chapter 7
Skill One: Cultivating Curiosity

1. Joseph Campbell, *The Power of Myth* (New York: Doubleday, 1988), 5.
2. Jiddu Krishnamurti, *On Fear* (San Francisco: HarperCollins, 1994).

3. Julia Cameron, *The Artist's Way: A Spiritual Path to Higher Creativity* (New York: Tarcher, 2002).

Chapter 8
Skill Two: Loving Ourselves from the Inside Out

1. ABC News, 20/20 *Downtown,* 2001.
2. Sri Nisargadatta Maharaj, *I Am That* (Bombay: Chetana Pvt., 1973), 8.
3. Jelaluddin Rumi, *The Love Poems of Rumi,* ed. Deepak Chopra (New York: Harmony Books, 1998), 39.
4. Pierre Teilhard de Chardin, quoted in *Simpson's Contemporary Quotations,* compiled by James B. Simpson (Boston: Houghton Mifflin, 1988), no. 4288.
5. Jon Kabat-Zinn, *Full Catastrophe Living: Using the Wisdom of Your Body and Mind to Face Stress, Pain, and Illness* (New York: Dell, 1990).
6. Thomas Merton, *Conjectures of a Guilty Bystander* (New York: Doubleday, 1965), 156.
7. Jack Kornfield, *A Grateful Heart,* ed. M. J. Ryan (Berkeley: Conari Press, 1994), 123.

Chapter 10
Skill Four: Coming Home to Ourselves

1. James Joyce, *Finnegans Wake* (New York: Penguin, 1999), quoted in Jack Kornfield, *A Path with Heart* (New York: Bantam, 1993), 43.
2. Quoted in Matthew Fox, *Sins of the Spirit, Blessings of the Flesh* (New York: Three Rivers Press, 1999), 29.
3. Fox, *Sins of the Spirit,* 48.
4. Jon Kabat-Zinn, *Full Catastrophe Living: Using the Wisdom of Your Body and Mind to Face Stress, Pain, and Illness* (New York: Dell, 1990), 216.

Notes

Chapter 11
Preparing to Find the Treasure

1. Gary Zukav, *The Seat of the Soul* (New York: Fireside, 1990). Interviewed on the *Oprah Winfrey Show*, December 6, 1999.

Chapter 14
Treasure Hunting with Feelings

1. Lynn Andrews, *Jaguar Woman* (San Francisco: HarperCollins, reprint, 1996), 14–15.
2. Thich Nhat Hanh, *Fragrant Palm Leaves* (Berkeley: Parallax Press, 1966), 109.

Chapter 15
Treasure Hunting with Compulsions

1. Eleanor Roosevelt, *You Learn by Living* (Louisville, KY: John Knox Press, 1983).

Appendix
Handy Reference Guide to Skills and Techniques

1. Antoine de Saint-Exupéry, *The Little Prince* (New York: Harcourt, 2000), 63.

Resources

Beck, Martha. *Expecting Adam: A True Story of Birth, Rebirth, and Everyday Magic.* New York: Berkley Publishing Group, 1999.

Hendricks, Gay. *Conscious Breathing: Breathwork for Health, Stress Release and Personal Mastery.* New York: Bantam Books, 1995.

Housden, Maria. *Hannah's Gift: Lessons from a Life Fully Lived.* New York: Bantam Books, 2002.

Johnson, Robert A. *Owning Your Own Shadow: Understanding the Dark Side of the Psyche.* San Francisco: HarperCollins, 1991.

Kabat-Zinn, Jon. *Full Catastrophe Living: Using the Wisdom of Your Body and Mind to Face Stress, Pain, and Illness.* New York: Dell Publishing, 1990.

Kornfield, Jack. *A Path with Heart: A Guide through the Perils and Promises of Spiritual Life.* New York: Bantam, 1993.

Kramer, Joel. *The Passionate Mind: A Manual for Living Creatively with One's Self.* Berkeley: North Atlantic Books, 1974.

Krishnamurti, J. *Freedom from the Known.* San Francisco: Harper-Collins, 1969.

Levine, Stephen. *Guided Meditations, Explorations, and Healings.* New York: Doubleday, 1991.

———. *Healing into Life and Death.* New York: Doubleday, 1987.

Muller, Wayne. *How Then Shall We Live? Four Simple Questions That Reveal the Beauty and Meaning of Our Lives.* New York: Bantam, 1996.

Ram Dass. *Grist for the Mill.* Santa Cruz, Calif.: Unity Press, 1977.

Roth, Geneen. *Feeding the Hungry Heart.* New York: Penguin, 1993.

————.*When Food Is Love: Exploring the Relationship between Eating and Intimacy.* New York: Penguin, 1992.

Swimme, Brian. *The Universe Is a Green Dragon: A Cosmic Creation Story.* Santa Fe, N.M.: Bear & Co., 1988.

Tolle, Eckhart. *The Power of Now: A Guide to Spiritual Enlightenment.* Novato, Calif.: New World Library, 1999.

Zukav, Gary. *The Heart of the Soul: Emotional Awareness.* New York: Simon & Schuster, 2002.

Index

Merton, Thomas, 137
mind, living in, 19–21, 168
mirrors, for seeing ourselves, 127, 138
mistakes, beating ourselves up for, 118
models, fashion, 168
Moody Blues, 265
movement, 184, 240–43, 268–69, 309–10

N

naming, power of. *See* "What am I experiencing?"
neck, feeling-generated sensations in, 227–28
needs. *See* "What do I *truly* need?"
negative vs. positive traits, 246–47
nervous system, 148, 239
nests for comfort, 185, 268–69
Nhat Hanh, Thich, 174, 247
no, empowered, 45, 153, 262–63, 288–92, 295, 300
num (healing force), 147

O

Odyssey (Homer), 193
opening the heart. *See* loving ourselves
opening to help, 214
opening to our breath. *See* breathing
overeating, 7–8, 185, 277, 281
oxygen, 147

P

pain
  breathing into, 149, 160, 165, 166

exercise, 180–81
meeting, 180–81
opening around vs. resisting, 165–66, 186
relief from, 134–35
types of, 180
parasympathetic nervous system, 148, 239
patience, 79–81, 86
Paul, the Apostle, 168
pause that refreshes, 176–77, 312
peace, 148–49
perfection, 20, 133–34, 142
Plato, 168–69
positive vs. negative traits, 246–47
prana (healing force), 147
presence to ourselves
  vs. being caught in our story, 264–65
  and compassion, 205
  through curiosity, 89–90, 107–8
  exercise, 107–8
  on the journey, 11–13
  through questions, 200
price of compulsions, 276–79
problems and solutions, 209
progress, 302

Q

questions, healing power of, 197–223
  breathing as enhancing, 238–39, 266–67
  check-in questions, 68–69, 105, 107–8, 179, 198, 199–207, 223, 308–9

330

About the Author

Mary O'Malley is an author, group facilitator, speaker, and counselor in private practice in Kirkland, Washington. For more than thirty years she has explored and practiced the art of being truly present to life, and out of this has evolved a system for awakening into the living moment of our lives, which she calls Awareness Meditation. Through her organization, Awakening, she invites others to find within a place of clarity, compassion, and trust they can access no matter what is happening. She extends an invitation to live from that place so that the impossible becomes possible and our hearts soar with the joy of being alive. Mary is available for speaking engagements, retreats, workshops, and phone and in-person counseling.

To contact Mary email her at awaken@maryomalley.com or go to her website: www.maryomalley.com.